A SOCIO-CULTURAL PERSPECTIVE ON PATIENT SAFETY

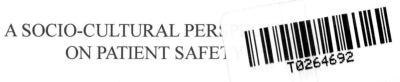

To err is human, to cover up is unforgivable,
and to fail to learn is inexcusable.

Sir Liam Donaldson,
World Alliance for Patient Safety,
27 October 2004

A Socio-cultural Perspective on Patient Safety

EDITED BY

EMMA ROWLEY
University of Nottingham, UK

&

JUSTIN WARING
Nottingham University Business School, UK

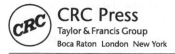

CRC Press
Taylor & Francis Group
Boca Raton London New York

CRC Press is an imprint of the
Taylor & Francis Group, an **informa** business

CRC Press
Taylor & Francis Group
6000 Broken Sound Parkway NW, Suite 300
Boca Raton, FL 33487-2742

First issued in paperback 2017

© 2011 by Emma Rowley and Justin Waring
CRC Press is an imprint of Taylor & Francis Group, an Informa business

No claim to original U.S. Government works

Version Date: 20160226

ISBN 13: 978-1-138-07281-7 (pbk)
ISBN 13: 978-1-4094-0862-8 (hbk)

Visit the Taylor & Francis Web site at
http://www.taylorandfrancis.com

and the CRC Press Web site at
http://www.crcpress.com

Contents

PART 4   KNOWLEDGE SHARING

PART 5   LEARNING

Author Biographies

Roland Bal is Professor of Healthcare Governance at the Institute of Health Policy and Management in Rotterdam, Netherlands. His research interests lie with the governance of health care, especially in terms of quality and safety.

Paul Barach is Visiting Professor the University of Utrecht in the Netherlands. He has over 15 years' experience in researching, teaching and applying human factors and quality improvement methods to health care and has been involved as a clinician, educator, researcher and policy-maker in enhancing health care improvement and patient safety policy in the United States, Europe and, more recently, in Australia.

Simon Bishop is lecturer in Organisational Behaviour at Nottingham University Business School. His research interests include work and employment in networked organisations; privatization and public–private partnerships; translating evidence to practice in health care; knowledge-sharing within and between organisations; health service reform and individual identity; qualitative and quantitative analysis of social networks and new managerial technologies in health care.

Graeme Currie is Professor of Public Management at Warwick Business School, UK. His work focuses on new organizational forms in health care; team-working in public services; knowledge management in health care and related industries and leadership in schools and health care organizations.

Anat Drach-Zahavy is a senior lecturer at the Faculty of Health and Welfare Sciences at the University of Haifa, Israel. She is the head of the research centre for the study, implementation and assimilation of evidence-based practice. Her research is in the areas of teamwork, safety and employee's health.

Rick Iedema is a Research Professor in Organizational Communication and Director at the Centre for Health Communication, Faculty of Arts and Social Sciences at the University of Technology, Sydney. His work addresses how the organization and communication of clinical work impact on patients' safety and well-being.

Jeanne Mengis is a senior research fellow at IKON and an Assistant Professor at the University of Lugano, Switzerland. In her research, she works on a communication perspective on knowledge processes in organizations and conducts research on cross-disciplinary collaboration, knowledge integration and evidence-based learning.

Jessica Mesman is senior lecturer at the Department of Technology and Society Studies at Maastricht University, Netherlands. Her ethnographic studies include investigations on neonatal intensive care units of what actually takes place at the interface of diagnosis and prognosis, of practitioners and technology, of medical facts and moral concerns.

Toby Murcott is a freelance science writer and journalist. Toby led the media analysis in the synthesis and narrative review of the UK's Patient Safety Research Portfolio outputs.

Davide Nicolini is joint Director of IKON and the Warwick Institute of Health, at Warwick Business School, UK. His work examines practice-based approaches to the study of knowing, learning and change in organizations; innovation process in health care and other complex environments; advancement of action-based approaches to learning and change and the study and promotion of safety.

Josephine Ocloo's background is in social work. Now specializing in patient safety, her research interests include medical harm, patient safety and empowering patients and the public in patient safety, tackling health inequalities, racism and broader areas of discrimination.

Cecily Palmer is a research fellow at University College London, UK. Cecily led the fieldwork and data analysis for a synthesis and narrative review of the research commissioned under the Patient Safety Research Portfolio (PSRP) – the UK's main source of funding for patient safety research. The review established principles to guide future patient safety research and investigated the wider impact of the PSRP research corpus.

Habibollah Pirnejad is Assistant Professor of Medical Informatics at the Urmia Medical Science University, Iran. He was a research fellow in Health Informatics at the Department of Health Policy and Management, Erasmus University Medical Center, Rotterdam, Netherlands. His research focuses on the application of information technology to improve communication and collaboration between health care professionals, especially concerning patient safety and workflow issues.

Emma Rowley is a senior research fellow at the University of Nottingham, UK. Emma's work combines theoretical arguments from medical sociology, science and technology studies and organizational studies in investigating the translation and utilization of innovative medical technologies in a number of health care contexts.

Of particular interest is how patient safety is negotiated when technologies and guidelines are introduced into practice.

Anit Somech is the head of Educational Leadership Department at the University of Haifa, Israel. Her research focuses on teamwork, management and work motivation.

Justin Waring is Professor of Health Systems and Policy at Nottingham University Business School. His research seeks to develop theoretical and methodological synthesis across social science disciplines to better understand clinical risk and organizational learning. This includes a study on the implementation of incident reporting, an ethnographic study of the threats to patient safety in the operating theatre, a real-time study of accident investigation, an evaluation of electronic prescribing in primary care and a mixed-methods study of learning across organizational and occupational boundaries in new clinical settings.

Foreword

Paul Barach

Visiting Professor, University of Utrecht, Netherlands

It seems that despite unprecedented levels of spending, preventable medical errors abound, uncoordinated care continues to frustrate patients and providers, and health care costs continue to rise. Although there has never been more awareness and resources devoted worldwide to overall system improvement, care experience, quality and safety, while advocating for system-wide culture change, there remain opportunities to achieve savings, reduce risks and improve performance. Current approaches are not producing the pace, breadth, or magnitude of improvement that patients demand and providers expect. Proscriptive rules, guidelines and checklists are helping to raise awareness and present some harm but are falling short from helping to provide an ultrasafe system (Amalberti et al. 2005). A new system centered around the patient and their clinical microsystem that renders clinical care processes more predictable, effective, efficient and humane is needed (Mohr et al. 2004).

These are the issues, among others, that concern Emma Rowley and Justin Waring, in their provocative book *A Socio-cultural Perspective on Patient Safety*. They come at the issues from different perspectives and are supported by an international cast of contributing cutting-edge thinkers. This stimulating book applies an interpretative social science lens to critically examine present thinking about how we can make health care safer and offer a complimentary perspective on how we move health care to higher reliability.

Mengis and Nicolini (Chapter 9 this volume) remind us that 'hospitals rarely learn from their mistakes' as providers do not feel safe to talk about their errors due to organizational secrecy that contributes to a lack of accountability and authentic communications. Why is the corporate culture of health care so secretive? Furthermore, routine nonconformity and socialization over many years can result in mistakes, misconduct and disaster (West 2000). The lack of psychological safety undermines safety practices, avoids tough conversations about the 'un-discussable', and keeps health care from becoming more reliable (Edmonson 1999). The cognitive dissonance that providers feel when confronted by organizational secrecy is predictable and leads to lack of information sharing, learning, and ultimately to disruptive behaviors, frustration and burnout.

At the heart of a sustainable, generative, continually improving health care system are three interlinked aims: (a) better outcomes (for example individuals, populations); b) better system performance (for example quality, safety, value); and (c) better professional development (for example competence, joy, pride)

(Batalden 2011). Rowley and Waring's bold vision for research and practice helps to move beyond the 'counting and control models' to one that addresses these aims, and supports dedicated workers struggling to manage the ever-growing complexity of their social–technical health care environments.

High reliability – or consistent performance at high levels of safety over long periods of time – is a hallmark for non-health, high-risk industries such as aviation and nuclear power (Weick et al. 2008). In the face of health reform and increased market competition, moving to high reliability requires adopting and supporting a culture of mindfulness in understanding the relationship and synergy of a variety of organizational risk factors and their effect on producing patient harm and inefficiency. This goes beyond rearranging the system's vulnerabilities but strives to understand how to support technology and learning that are embedded in practice, and encourages norms and values of high reliability organizations: preoccupation with failure; reluctance to simplify operations, commitment to resilience and deference to sharp end, front line users.

Moreover, the available evidence suggests that the risk of harmful error in health care may be increasing in spite of the important work of the last decade. Regulatory and standard-setting bodies around the world are all very clear about the need for more accountability and mindfulness, real patient focus and empowerment and enhanced value in all domains. A variety of strategies are beginning to be employed throughout the health care industry to address the central issue of value and enhanced resilience, with the goal of improving the net ratio of benefits obtained per dollar spent on health care. Enhancing safety, quality and value in health care will require listening and being responsive to stakeholder perspectives, starting with the patient, their families and the informal clinician collaboratives of practice. Lessons from high-reliability science and past efforts to improve health care quality point to the importance of leadership commitment, full implementation of a safety culture and thorough adoption of robust process improvement tools and methods while identifying the key barriers and outlining the opportunities for engagement.

Collective mindfulness means that everyone who works in health care is accountable and becomes acutely aware that even small failures in safety protocols or processes can lead to catastrophic adverse outcomes. As a matter of routine, workers in these organizations are always searching for the smallest indication that the environment or a key safety process goal has drifted or changed in some way that might lead to failure, if some action is not taken to solve the problem (de Wilde 2000). Continuously uncovering these safety concerns will permit providers and their organizations to identify safety or quality problems at a stage when they are easily fixed. In health care we are too often in the position of investigating adverse events using rigid tools such as root cause analysis after the patient has been injured, which means that we have missed opportunities to pinpoint and correct quality problems before they cause harm. When incident investigations are de-coupled from practice, and are poorly reconciled with the practical, material and temporal arrangements of delivering health care service they miss the organizational, political and emotional processes of learning. Perhaps we need to be studying the latent competencies (exnovation) that offer insights into the ability of clinicians to produce reliable and safe outcomes despite the complexity of their day-to-day practice (Mesman 2010)?

In addition to the overarching atmosphere of collective mindfulness, high-reliability organizations have two other features in common. First, after organizations identify potential deficiencies in safety processes, they eliminate these deficiencies through the use of robust process improvement methodologies that are led by users and based on their wisdom and heuristics to improve their processes. Second, the organizations rely on a particular organizational culture to ensure the performance of improved safety processes over long periods of time and to remain constantly aware of the possibility of failure and normalized deviance, in which risk can become normalized within the prevailing culture (Vaughan 1999). This may be called a safety culture.

Trust has heavily eroded in health care leading to cynicism and disengagement. Trust-building measures are essential in two different ways if health care is to receive a continuous flow of information about possible hazards, near misses or unsafe conditions. First, all front-line workers (clinical and administrative) must trust each other in order to feel safe when they identify a problem that may involve or uncover errors made by others. Living systems adapt and respond to their internal and external contexts. Without trust, they resist intentional change partly because there are competing commitments and assumptions that effectively hold the unchanged present in place.

Improvement requires bringing multiple knowledge systems together. What Rowley and Waring's provocative book posits is that generalizable social science in a particular context supported by measured performance improvement together could help make health care more resilient. 'Good' science involves more than evidence of effect and requires innovative research methods including action research, expansive learning and other ethno-methodologies. These new methods can help shed light on the relationships and interactions between health care providers, patients and the technologies that support this interaction. The shared benefit of these methods can lead to active entanglement of patients, providers and the research community working together, using storytelling, videos and personal reflections to engender respect, trust and collaborative relationships.

Complexity science teaches us that there are three types of problems that we face in the world: simple (for example, baking a cake); complicated (for example, riding a bicycle); complex (for example, raising a child) (Glouberman and Zimmerman 2002). In complex settings (for example, patient handovers, managing deteriorating patients) where the elements and interactions are not knowable, and although there is a shared aim, and relationships among the team members matter, reliability may not be possible and we must train and expect growing degrees of resilience as a more realistic aim.

Ackoff wrote about 'power over' versus 'power to' get things done (Ackoff et al. 2006). 'Power over' is the exercise of authority, to punish or reward. 'Power to' is the force of ideas to inspire, engage and transform front line workers into champions of these change ideas. As the health workforce increases in its knowledge of systems, reliability and relational value, the success of health organizations shifts from 'power over' workers and patients to 'power to', from top-down management to a partnership–leadership model, starting with the patient and their family. While there is little question that quality improvement and patient safety lies at the heart of a major shift in how people think about and execute health care delivery, it is a massive transformation that will span a full generation. The ideas in this book could not be more timely. It presents a road map and a 'how to think differently' about how best to engage patients and health care providers emotionally and intellectually in health care transformation that is the core work of this generation of caring professionals.

References

Ackoff, R., Magidison, J. and Addison, H. 2006. *Idealized Design: How to Dissolve Tommorow's Crisis Today*. Upper Saddle River, New Jersey: Wharton School Publishing.

Amalberti, R., Auroy, Y., Berwick, D.M. and Barach, P. 2005. Five system barriers to achieving ultra-safe health care. *Annals of Internal Medicine*, 142(9), 756–64.

Batalden, P. 2011. *Leading the Improvement of Health Care 'A one page book'*. 18 May 2011. Available at http://tdi.dartmouth.edu/documents/Batalden%20 1%20page%20book.pdf.

Carroll, J. 1998. Organizational learning activities in high-hazard industries: the logics underlying self-analysis. *Journal of Management Studies*, 35(6), 699–717.

Edmonson, A. 1999. Psychological safety and learning behaviours in work teams. *Administrative Science Quarterly*, 44(2), 350–83.

Glouberman, S. and Zimmerman, B. 2002. *Complicated and Complex Systems: What Would Successful Reform of Medicare Look Like? Discussion paper no. 8*. Saskatoon: Commission on the Future of Health Care in Canada.

Mesman, J. 2010. Diagnostic work in collaborative practices in neonatal care. In: *Ethnographies of Diagnostic work: Dimensions of Transformative Practice*, edited by M. Büscher, D. Goodwin, and J. Mesman. Basingstoke: Palgrave Macmillan, pp. 95–112.

Mohr, J., Batalden, P. and Barach, P. 2004. Integrating patient safety into the clinical microsystem, *Quality and Safety in Healthcare*, 13, 34–8.

Vaughan, D. 1999. The dark side of organizations: mistake, misconduct and disaster. *Annual Review of Sociology*, 25, 271–305.

Weick, K., Sutcliffe, K. and Obstfeld, D. 2008. Organizing for high reliability: processes of collective mindfulness. In: *Crisis Management*, edited by A. Boin. Thousand Oaks, CA: Sage, pp. 31–67.

West, E. 2000. Organisational sources of safety and danger: sociological contributions to the study of adverse events. *Quality in Health Care*, 9, 120–6.

Wilde de, R. 2000. Innovating Innovation: a contribution to the philosophy of the future. Keynote speech at Policy Agendas for Sustainable Technological Innovation, London.

Introduction:
A Socio-cultural Perspective on Patient Safety

Emma Rowley and Justin Waring

Over twenty or so years, the movement to enhance patient safety has gone from a slow burning fuse to a worldwide explosion of activity. In its early years, the patient safety movement (if it could be termed a movement at this time) was concerned to highlight and determine the existence and nature of the safety problems facing health care systems. The landmark Harvard Medical Practice study, for instance, estimated the degree and character of iatrogenic illness within the USA brought about by adverse clinical events (Brennan et al. 1991, Leape et al. 1991). In many ways, error and harm were largely marginal to mainstream health services research and health care policies. However, it is important to note that these issues had been the focus of several social science research studies (Hughes 1951, Freidson 1970, Millman 1976, Bosk 1979, Paget 1988). By the later 1990s, almost a decade after the seminal Harvard study, a sea-change occurred. Heightened awareness of patient safety was created through the publication of the USA's *To Err is Human* (Institute of Medicine 1999), the UK's *An Organization with a Memory* (Department of Health 2000), New Zealand's *Review of the Processes Concerning Adverse Medical Events* (Cull 2001), and Australia's *Iatrogenic Injury in Australia* (Runciman and Moller 2001). All of these reports placed patient safety firmly on the health policy agenda, and led to a growing field of learning and research in patient safety. Since this time research and policy has matured to better understand why threats to safety come about and how learning from these events can best be turned into systemic service improvement.

At the heart of the global patient safety agenda is a commitment to the principle of 'first, do no harm'. The agenda recognizes that, despite the best intentions and efforts of health care professionals, mistakes will happen. Consideration has turned, therefore, to understanding more about the fundamentals of human error and the ways in which 'honest mistakes' can be avoided or their effects mitigated. It is at this juncture that policymakers and have turned to the experiences of industries such as aviation, space travel, nuclear power, shipping and petrochemicals that are not only high risk, but consistently shown to be reliable in terms of how they manage the risks to safety and promote organizational learning. In seeking to emulate these industries, the patient safety movement therefore embraced the principles of 'safety science', including the theoretical and practical contributions from cognitive and social psychology, ergonomics and human factors and strategic risk management (Sheen 1987, Weick 1990, Leape 1997, Helmreich 2000, NASA/Columbia Accident Investigation Board 2003, Woods and Cook 2003, Starbuck and Farjoun 2005). These have helped to redefine our understanding of patient safety by highlighting a distinction between the 'active errors' inherent within human behaviour and the underlying 'latent' factors that condition or make possible these mistakes. Often illustrated as the Swiss Cheese Model (Reason 1997), analytical attention is therefore redirected to the sequence and contribution of upstream and contextual factors that make human error almost an inevitable feature of organizational life, including for example the design of tasks, communication flows, team working arrangements, warning systems and the management of resources.

These ideas have informed the development and application of practical techniques and procedures to better identify and learn from past mistakes and service failures. Although these practices vary in detail between individual health care systems, they share a common aim to improve the safety of patient care through introducing systems for organizational learning that capture information about clinical risks, so as to facilitate the discovery and control of factors that enable or exacerbate the potential for human error. As with other forms of strategic risk management, this is often premised on the creation of procedures for knowledge sharing, such as incident reporting, which allow for front line events and risk(s) to be communicated more widely with colleagues. Through the collection of this information it is then possible for service providers to systematically look across clinical risks, investigate the underlying factors, and instigate change so as to protect staff and patients from recurrence. Again, borrowing from other high-risk industries, this is sometimes described as *root cause analysis*, which involves a structured and systematic analysis of the latent factors that contributed to unsafe practice.

Policymakers understand, however, that there are many barriers to the management of safety. Perhaps the most significant of these relates to the reluctance of staff to participate in incident reporting. This is conventionally attributed to a 'blame culture' within health care, which discourages staff from being open and honest about their mistakes in the belief that they will be reprimanded or disciplined. This assignment of individual blame reflects a 'person-centred' view of safety that is ignorant of the latent factors, whilst emphasizing the need to instil a 'just culture' that fosters openness without the fear of blame (Reason 1997). More broadly speaking, the creation of a 'safety culture' is seen as fundamental to the success of safety management, which involves shared attitudes, beliefs and practices related to safety, including mindfulness to danger; appreciation of the 'systems approach'; openness, trust and the sharing of information; a reflexive attitude towards safety improvement; and effective leadership that promotes the goals of safety. Again, such a culture is typical of other high-risk, high reliability organizations, and is often promoted as a panacea to the management of patient safety (Helmreich and Merritt 1998, Weick 1991).

Drawing on the theories of safety science and the experiences of other high-risk industries, the global patient safety movement is therefore characterized by the articulation of a new way of thinking about safety that follows the principles of human factors, the implementation of new risk management procedures to learn from past experiences of unsafe patient care, together with the modification of staff attitudes and cultures so as to support the implementation of change.

Supporting the roll-out and implementation of the patient safety agenda, considerable research has been undertaken to understand more about the fundamentals of safety and risk within health care: Lilford (2010) on the sources of danger in medicating, Helmreich and Davies (1996) on risks within the operating theatre, Tighe et al. (2006) on the threats to safety in Accident and Emergency departments. Research has also been undertaken to examine the best techniques for adapting and applying human factors-type approaches in health care, for example how to transfer the principles of crew resource management developed in the aviation sector to the acute hospital (Morey et al. 2002) or how to undertake root cause analysis (JCAHO 2000). Studies have also been conducted to further understand how organizational cultures impact upon patient safety, for example developing tools to characterize and measure safety cultures in primary care and secondary care (Pronovost and Sexton 2005, Kirk et al. 2005). In addition, studies have examined the best ways to implement incident reporting and encourage staff participation, for example through undertaking comparative analysis of different health care sectors and other industries (Helmreich and Merritt 1998).

Although such research, like policy, is driven by the desire to improve the quality and safety of patient care, it is often unquestioning and uncritical of the prevailing policy orthodoxy, typically seeking to endorse and facilitate its implementation. In being uncritical, research can sometimes appear myopic, failing to ask questions about the underlying nature of the problem, such as the institutional and political imperatives underlying risk, or being overly simplistic in transferring solutions found in other sectors, such as crew resource management, whilst also being negligent of the knock-on effects of change, for example, in professional practices and identity. This book describes, analyses and critiques the assumptions that ground the contemporary patient safety movement, the policy orthodoxy that it embraces and the technocratic solutions it produces.

Whilst the prevailing conceptual and theoretical orthodoxy around patient safety acknowledges the multifaceted nature of the problem, and without question seeks to change health care services for the better, it is characterized and underpinned by a 'measure and manage' approach to safety. As such, policies, research and management tend to define and respond to the problem of patient safety in a way that can gloss over the complexities of health care organization and delivery, including the socio-cultural fabric of organization and occupational life, and the wider historical, political and institutional context of health service delivery. For example, in approaching the notion of 'culture' research has tended towards the development of tools that can measure cultural attributes along predefined dimensions that are believed to relate to safety as a basis for making connections between culture and performance and for directing management intervention. However, questions need to be asked whether the cultural context of safety is easily amenable to such measurement and change. Other studies in the social sciences, particularly anthropology and sociology, tell us that cultures are deeply held complex systems of shared and often tacit meanings and values that are acquired through many years of socialization and inform social action, identity and belonging. As such it is often difficult to accurately 'capture' such qualities through predefined measures and they are typically difficult to change. Moreover, when seeking to identify the sources of risk that threaten safety, the logic of safety science and human factors directs us to identify the latent factors that threaten safety, but how far or deep should this analysis develop and at which level should it cease? For example, should we be asking questions merely about the organization of clinical tasks or should we be focusing on broader questions about occupational relationships or the political priorities that frame the allocation and management of health care resources? Furthermore, much work has been directed at developing and defining a standardized taxonomy of clinical error, but such work fails to acknowledge that the perception, interpretation and definition of error varies between occupational groups and organizational contexts, being framed by the wider socio-cultural context and representing complex expressions of social power and control.

At the level of reform and quality improvement, policies tend to borrow and modify concepts, models and practices applied in other industries. These are often presented as the simple solutions to patient safety, but few people question the merits or appropriateness of transferring and applying those strategies, techniques and methods developed in aviation or nuclear energy, or the possibility of developing more fruitful courses of action. Returning again to the example of culture discussed above, what we see is a single-minded approach that is based upon and reinforces the view that culture exists as an entity or variable that can and should be managed, with a direct, identifiable impact on safety outcomes. Such endeavours often fail to be deterred by the increasing weight of evidence that suggests the limitations of such approaches in bringing about real benefit, and that the nature of the problem might be more complex than accounted for. More broadly the vast majority of research in the area of patient safety has ignored or paid insufficient attention the rich legacy of social science that deals directly with the issues of clinical error and risk. Of particular note is Bosk's (1979) ethnographic account of surgical training that explores how mistakes at work are 'forgiven' but 'remembered' in the social routines and rituals that comprise professional socialization. Moreover, Paget's (1988) phenomenological account of how doctors react to safety events highlights the important, but largely neglected, emotional dimension. More recently, Rosenthal (1995) revealed the deeply engrained social and cultural practices that frame the collegial efforts in managing poor performance.

Overall, this mainstream or orthodox patient safety approach can be thought of as the dominant paradigm. It has become the frame of reference for understanding and approaching the problem of patient safety. It has become embedded and taken for granted in health policies and health service research to the extent that other, more critical perspectives remain marginal. If we are really serious about patient safety, however, we need to look beyond the the solutions currently being presented and seek to both understand and engage with the complexities of the socio-cultural and political context of health care organization and delivery. Mainstream patient safety has a tendency to be narrow and presumptuous, portraying health care practices as simplistic. In doing so, it dangerously ignores the local specificities and complexities that create threats to patient safety.

Much of the literature on organizational learning points us to the barriers of implementing top-down forms of knowledge management, as well as to the fact that knowledge is shared through interaction and learning situated in context and practice (Lave and Wenger 1991). It is critical, therefore, to understand more about the socio-cultural, organizational and political context of safety and learning. Consequently, this book is an attempt to examine and question the orthodox assumptions found in policy and mainstream patient safety research. We suggest an alternative conceptualization of the patient safety domain, in terms of how the problem is defined, the questions asked and what might constitute the means of addressing them. This involves viewing socio-cultural and political issues as central to patient safety. It requires a widening of our analytic lens, utilizing theories and methodologies that embrace this complexity to examine aspects of health care that are often overlooked within mainstream research.

This edited collection brings together researchers from around the world who are examining the facets of health care organization and delivery that are sometimes marginal to mainstream patient safety theories and methodologies. These somewhat neglected areas offer important insights into the socio-cultural and organizational context of patient safety. The chapters offer a more critical appreciation of patient safety in comparison to the current orthodox approach to patient safety and clinical risk, which has a tendency to neglect or downplay important issues associated with professional practice, teamwork, culture and organizational complexity. Given that patient safety remains a growing area of research and policy, we feel it is important to offer a more nuanced and complex interpretation of the problem and the policy responses. Through examining these critical insights or perspectives and drawing upon theories and methodologies often neglected by mainstream safety researchers, we can understand more, not simply about the barriers and drivers to implementing patient safety programmes, but also about the more fundamental issues that shape notions of safety, alternate strategies for enhancing safety and the wider implications of the safety agenda on the future of health care delivery. Consequently, this book exposes the taken for granted assumptions around fundamental philosophical and political issues upon which mainstream patient safety orthodoxy relies.

The collection draws upon a range of theoretical and empirical approaches from across the social sciences to investigate and question the patient safety movement. Each chapter takes as its focus and question a particular aspect of the patient safety reforms, from its policy context and theoretical foundations to its practical application and manifestation in clinical practice, whilst also considering the wider implications for the organization and delivery of health care services. The book is structured into five sections, each critically examining patient safety in relation to (1) patients and publics, (2) clinical practice, (3) technology, (4) knowledge sharing, and (5) learning.

The collection opens with two chapters that address a largely forgotten or overlooked area, which represents a massive gap in terms of thinking about how safety events and research are communicated to the public, and how the public should be involved in safety events. Palmer and Murcott's chapter offers a critical examination of patient safety in the media. They describe a paradox in the media's representation and portrayal of patient safety, pointing out that only 'bad news' stories such as high profile incidents are reported. In contrast, they argue that the work and effort that goes into protecting patient safety is relatively ignored, as it is not considered to be 'newsworthy' (in terms of selling newspapers). This consequently creates a tension between the researchers and practitioners creating good patient safety stories, and the mass media. Ocloo draws our attention to another disturbing gap in the patient safety literature. She explores the role and the voice of patients in patient safety, by looking back at the development of user involvement in UK health policy and health social movements.

Mainstream approaches to patient safety offer something of a paradoxical view of clinical practice. On the one hand, efforts have been made to depict safe working practices as being framed not by individual factors, but wider upstream factors. On the other hand, much attention has been directed at improving safe practice, through better communication, diagnostic skills, checklists etc. (rather than system-level improvements). In the chapters in this section of the collection, practice is deconstructed and presented in a way that highlights the hidden or neglected competencies that make clinical practice safe. Drach-Zahavy and Somech discuss the gap between policy and practice, by examining nurses' decision-making and use of heuristics in rationalizing their actions. They suggest that non-adherence to rules and guidelines is not something that occurs in an ad hoc fashion, but is systematic and predictable. Mesman continues this focus on the minutiae of health care practice, focusing on what makes safe practice (opposed to what causes errors). She finds that safety is produced, and is a form of medicine-in-action.

The collection's next section reminds us that technology and design are not necessarily the safety solution so often presented in policies. In particular, we note the almost taken for granted assumption that technological innovation, especially ICTs, will enhance safe decision-making, prescribing and dispensing, surgical and anaesthetic safety or provide the basis for organizational learning. The chapters presented in this collection, however, reveal a different picture where technologies are far from being a safety fix. Like the preceding chapter by Mesman, Rowley's chapter is also an example of medicine-in-practice, exploring the use of medical devices. Concentrating on single use devices, she asks if breaking medical device rules should always result in a patient safety incident, or if breaking the rules – acting deviantly – can actually protect patients. Pirnejad and Bal's chapter focuses on the threats to patient safety linked to information technology systems utilized in medication administration. Drawing on a wide variety of data, they explore how information technology can create threats to safety through interoperability problems, dissociation between the virtual and real world, and workflow impediments.

Underpinning much of the patient safety research and practice is an assumption that improved learning results in part from enhanced communication and knowledge sharing. This can be seen with the emphasis given to incident reporting and other initiatives to enhance communication, such as the use of checklists. Although there is frequent mention of the barriers to communication, such as culture or status differentials, there remains little detailed appreciation of how, when and why clinicians communicate in practice and how they respond to current initiatives to improve communication. The chapters presented in this section of the collection explore this knowledge-sharing gap. Waring and Currie investigate how different groups of medical professionals interact with the UK's National Reporting and Learning System (NRLS), which records all patient safety incidents and near-misses that individuals take the time to report. They suggest that the NRLS can be a source of conflict, and echo the tensions between managers and doctors. Using social network analysis, Bishop and Waring's chapter explores how professional-practice networks can contribute to patient safety through an examination of knowledge sharing and information flows between and across health care professions.

Central to the safety agenda is the idea that learning will inevitably lead to service improvement. This follows a model of learning which is largely linear and abstract, and importantly unlike other more situated models of action learning. The last section of our collection investigates the concept of learning-in-practice in more detail. Mengis and Nicolini's chapter explores the use of root cause analysis (RCA) to investigate lessons from clinical adverse events. They critique how RCA can lead to organizational learning, through investigating the cause(s) of incidents, by looking at how the use of RCA was played out in context. Finally, Iedema examines the influence of changing contexts and dynamics in health care, and argues for a real-time, *in situ* understanding of and response to medical errors, harms and bad practice. He calls for a new knowledge to be developed, incorporating formal knowledge and awareness of *in situ* complexities.

Taken as a whole, the book advances a strong, coherent argument that is much needed to counter some of the uncritical assumptions that need to be described and analysed if patient safety is, indeed, to be achieved.

References

Bosk, C. 1979. *Forgive and Remember: Managing Medical Mistakes*. Chicago, IL: Chicago University Press.

Brennan, T.A., Leape, L.L., Laird, N.M., Hebert, L., Localio, A.R., Lawthers, A.G., Newhouse, J.P., Weiler, P.C. and Hiatt, H.H. 1991. Incidence of adverse events and negligence in hospitalized patients. Results of the Harvard Medical Practice Study I. *New England Journal of Medicine*, 324(6), 370–6.

Cull, H. 2001. *Review of the Processes Concerning Adverse Medical Events*. Wellington: Ministry of Health.

Department of Health. 2000. *An Organization with a Memory*. London: The Stationery Office.

Donaldson, L. 2004. *World Alliance for Patient Safety*. Washington, DC, 27 October 2004.

Freidson, E. 1970. *The Profession of Medicine*. New York: Harper Row.

Helmreich, R.L. and Davies, J.M. 1996. Human factors in the operating room: interpersonal determinants of safety, efficiency and morale. In: *Quality Assurance and Risk Management in Anaesthesia. Clinical Anaesthesiology: International Practice and Research* 10(2), edited by Alan Aitkenhead. London: Balliére, pp. 277–98.

Helmreich, R. and Merrit, A. 1998. *Culture at Work in Aviation and Medicine*. Aldershot: Ashgate.

Helmreich, R.L. 2000. On error management: lessons from aviation. *British Medical Journal,* 320, 781–5.

Hughes, E.C. 1951. Mistakes at work. *Canadian Journal of Economics and Political Science*, 17(3), 320–7.

Institute of Medicine. 1999. *To Err is Human: Building A Safer Health System*. Washington, DC: National Academy Press.

JCAHO (Joint Commission on Accreditation of Healthcare Organizations). 2000. *Root Cause Analysis in Health Care: Tools and Techniques*. Oakbrook Terrace, IL: Joint Commission on Accreditation of Health Care Organizations.

Kirk, S., Marshall, M., Claridge, T., Esmail, A. and Parker, D. 2005. Evaluating safety culture. In: *Patient Safety: Research into Practice*, edited by Kieran Walshe and Ruth Boaden. Milton Keynes: Open University Press, pp. 173–84.

Lave, J. and Wenger, E. 1991. *Situated Learning – Legitimate Peripheral Participation*. Cambridge: Cambridge University Press.

Leape, L.L., Brennan, T.A., Laird, N. Lawthers, A.G., Localio, A.R., Barnes, B.A., Hebert, L., Newhouse, J.P., Weiler, P.C. and Hiatt, H. 1991. The nature of adverse events in hospitalized patients. Results of the Harvard Medical Practice Study II. *New England Journal of Medicine*, 324(6), 377–84.

Leape, L.L. 1997. A systems analysis to medical error. *Journal of Evaluation in Clinical Practice*, 3(3), 213–22.

Lilford, R. 2010. The English Patient Safety Research Programme: a commissioner's tale. *Journal of Health Services Research and Policy*, 15(s1), 1–3.

Millman, M. 1976. *The Unkindest Cut: Life in the Backrooms of Medicine*. New York: Morrow.

Morey, J.C., Simon, R., Jay, G.D., Wears, R.L., Salisbury, M., Dukes, K.A. and Burns, S.D. 2002. Error reduction and performance improvement in the emergency department through formal teamwork training: evaluation results of the MedTeams Project. *Health Services Research*, 37(6), 1553–81.

NASA/Columbia Accident Investigation Board. 2003. *Report Volume 1*. Washington, DC: Government Printing Office.

Paget, M.A. 1988. *The Unity of Mistakes: A Phenomenological Interpretation of Medical Work*. Philadelphia, PA: Temple University Press.

Pronovost, P. and Sexton, B. 2005. Assessing safety culture: guidelines and recommendations. *Qaulity and Safety in Healthcare*, 14, 231–223.

Reason, J. 1997. *Managing the Risks of Organizational Accidents*. Aldershot: Ashgate.

Rosenthal, M. 1995. *The Incompetent Doctor*. Maidenhead: Open University Press.

Runciman, W.B. and Moller, J. 2001. *Iatrogenic Injury in Australia*. Adelaide: Australian Patient Safety Foundation.

Sheen, Mr Justice. 1987. *MV Herald of Free Enterprise. Report of Court No. 8074 Formal Investigation*. London: Department of Transport.

Starbuck, W.H. and Farjoun, M. 2005. *Organization at the Limit: Lessons from the Columbia Disaster*. Oxford: Blackwell.

Tighe, C.M., Woloshynowych, M., Brown, R., Wears, B. and Vincent, C. 2006. Incident reporting in one UK accident and emergency department. *Accident and Emergency Nursing*, 14(1), 27–37.

Weick, K.E. 1990. The vulnerable system: an analysis of the Tenerife air disaster. *Journal of Management*, 16(3), 571–93.

Weick, K. 1991. Organizational culture as a source of high reliability. *California Management Review*, 29, 112–17.

Woods, D.D. and Cook, R.I. 2003. Mistaking error. In: *Patient Safety Handbook*, edited by Martin Hatlie and Barbara Youngberg. Sudbury: Jones and Bartlett Publishers, pp. 95–108.

PART 1
Patients and Publics

Chapter 1

'All News is Bad News':
Patient Safety in the News Media

Cecily Palmer and Toby Murcott

This chapter explores the paradox of patient safety in the media: put simply, deficiencies in patient safety receive ample coverage, whereas the improvement and maintenance of patient safety receive far less. We present and reflect on the findings of a media impact assessment undertaken as part of a review of the UK-based programme of patient safety research: the Patient Safety Research Portfolio (PSRP). The assessment sought to identify and examine coverage of PSRP-funded patient safety research studies in the UK news media. We found only a single news story that referenced a PSRP study, even though 27 of the studies were complete at the time of our review. By contrast, stories covering serious or fatal patient safety incidents, strategies for improving patient safety in their aftermath and calls to improve patient safety made by those affected by such incidents were a regular feature in the UK news media at the time.

Existing studies of health and illness stories in the media have focused on coverage of patient safety failures in hospitals and health care settings, which frequently garner huge media attention (Stebbing and Kaushal 2006). Examples of incidents to have received major coverage in the UK news media include severe failings in emergency care involving Mid-Staffordshire NHS Foundation Trust and the death of a young man after the leukaemia drug Vincristine was mistakenly injected into his spine. Millenson (2002) argues that, though research on medical errors leading to the harm of patients had been published in the US context, this had led to little change in medical practice. He further claims that extensive media coverage of errors and fatal mistakes made by health professionals forced the profession to acknowledge this problem, and begin to establish organizations and develop the expertise necessary to prevent medical errors. Consistent with Millenson's argument, the exposure and investigation of care failings at Mid-Staffordshire NHS Foundation Trust was preceded by sustained media coverage of the campaign started by Julie Bailey, whose mother died at the hospital due to 'appalling emergency care' (Healthcare Commission 2009). It can therefore be argued that media coverage of patient safety failures has played an important role in prompting professional and governmental responses to patient safety failures in health care settings.

This chapter will focus on the absence of patient safety success stories in the media, as illustrated by our investigation of media coverage of the PSRP research corpus, and attempt to explain why so few positive or hopeful patient safety stories were found in the media coverage. This omission is despite the existence of a considerable programme of research dedicated to investigating and improving patient safety. Having illustrated the paradox of patient safety in the media – that patient safety receives coverage when failing or deficient, whereas positive patient safety stories are largely absent, this chapter considers and reflects on the tension that has traditionally characterized the relationship between research communities and the mass media. It concludes with a strategy that patient safety researchers and research commissioners might use to address the imbalance in coverage of patient safety issues and research.

Assessing 'Impact': Search Strategy for News Media Coverage of the PSRP Studies

The PSRP was founded in June 2001 with the aim of identifying processes and structures that might reduce the probability of adverse clinical events and evaluating interventions seeking to change the health care system and improve patient safety (Lilford et al. 2005: 3). The PSRP commissioned 36 diverse, multidisciplinary research studies undertaken between 2001 and 2009[1] that examined and critically reflected upon the risks to the safety of patients; structures and processes that minimize such risks; and interventions with the potential to improve the overall safety of the NHS. We were part of the research team commissioned in 2008 to produce a narrative review of completed PSRP research studies that would summarize and synthesize the findings of the corpus (see Dingwall et al. 2009).

Part of the review assessed the impact of the PSRP research corpus in terms of coverage in both popular news media and specialist medical publications. Four approaches were used to determine the degree of coverage of patient safety research portfolio studies. Searches of Nexis, the comprehensive print news database, were used to identify UK local and national print news media coverage that could be directly linked or attributed to any of the PSRP studies. Full project titles were used as the primary search term and this was followed by searches using keywords from the titles of the studies. If 50 or fewer hits were located by the search, these were checked manually for references to the PSRP projects. If more than 50 hits were returned by the search, secondary searches were performed on the subset using the name of the relevant principal investigator, and separately, the names of study co-authors. In all cases an assessment of whether a story was linked or attributable to a PSRP study was made by reading the story in full and searching for specific references to the study, to the institution in which the study was undertaken and/or to the principal or co-investigators on the study.

---

1   The PSRP research corpus is available at http://www.haps.bham.ac.uk/publichealth/ psrp/commissioned.shtml.

A common criticism of medical and scientific communication studies is that 'researchers studying media' are in fact 'researchers study[ing] newspapers' (Gregory and Miller 1998: 105), and we therefore endeavoured also to include the outputs of non-textual broadcast media in our search strategy. We searched the websites of three major UK broadcast media agencies (BBC, ITN and Sky) for both audiovisual and text-based articles making reference to the PSRP projects. Each website was searched, using the full title of each PSRP research study and the names of the principal investigators and co-investigators as search terms. Hits located using the searches were checked manually for references or links to the PSRP study in question. These searches located no news stories that could be directly linked to any of the studies in the PSRP corpus of research.[2]

Our search of academic and professional publications covered four journals selected because of their relevance to health care professionals in the UK. Due to there being no central database for the large range of professional publications relevant to health care professionals in the UK, the pragmatic decision was made to search the archives of the *British Medical Journal* news section, *The Lancet* news section, the *Nursing Times* and the *Health Services Research Journal* for coverage of the PSRP studies. Our searches of these publications, using the same terms outlined above, located no stories that could be directly attributed to the PSRP corpus of research.

The press release archives from the home institutions of each principal investigator of a PSRP study were also searched to determine whether any of the institutions hosting PSRP research had produced related press releases. Our search relied on the online press release archives that are publicly accessible via most university websites, including the Universities of York, Newcastle, Nottingham, Manchester, Imperial College London, Salford, Dundee, Bristol, UCL and other institutions involved in 21 of the PSRP studies. We located just one press release about a PSRP study being undertaken at the University of Nottingham; however it did not appear to have contributed to an identifiable story in the popular media.

Finally, to get a broader sense of patient safety stories that occurred in UK newspaper coverage within the time frame of the PSRP research studies, we also searched the Nexis database using a small group of keywords that were common to much of the reporting of patient safety issues. These searches, which included the terms 'e-prescribing', 'medication errors' and 'checklists', were performed in order to produce a brief, pragmatic review of the type of story published in the popular media with reference to patient safety.

Our searches of the Nexis database for coverage of PSRP studies located a single story that was directly linked to a PSRP study. Published in *The Times* on 21 May 2003 (Wright 2003), the story covered the introduction of 'aviation-style near-miss reports for family doctors' and made reference to the findings of a

---

2   We acknowledge that these websites are not maintained as a comprehensive or authoritative database of the content or coverage of their respective news organizations and accept that this is a limitation of our search strategy.

specific PSRP study which examined the nature and frequency of medical errors in primary care (Sandars and Esmail 2001); it further included a number of quotes from the principal investigator of the study:

> Doctors know from their own experience that things go wrong ... often nothing happens as a result and there is no real harm done ... what we don't have is an accurate idea of the scale of the problem. In the past studies have tended to look at medical errors in hospitals and not primary care (Esmail, quoted in Wright 2003).

As news stories often evolve rapidly away from their original inspiration or stimulus without leaving an identifiable trail of facts or sources from which they originally derived, it is possible that further stories based on research from the PSRP corpus were not identified using this search strategy and we acknowledge this as a potential limitation to our work.

Categories of Patient Safety Story in the News Media

To summarize, our investigation of different media for coverage of the PSRP research studies, which incorporated searches of the websites of the major UK broadcast media agencies, of professional publications relevant to UK health practitioners, of university press release archives and of the Nexis print media database, located a single news story that could be directly linked to a research study within the PSRP corpus. While we only located a single story related to PSRP, our searches revealed that a variety of topics related to patient safety were featured at some length, especially in the UK newspapers. Our searches for the terms 'electronic prescribing' and 'medication errors' generated a number of hits on both the BBC website and in the Nexis database. The pragmatic review of patient safety stories using additional searches of the Nexis database found that patient safety issues featured regularly in the UK news media, and that this coverage could be separated into three broad categories.

The principal category of patient safety story referred to specific cases of safety failure in which a serious or fatal incident had occurred. The source for this type of story was typically an official announcement from the hospital or Trust at which the incident had occurred, as apparent in the following example:

> Heartache for family over boy's leukaemia medicine blunder. Hospital bosses have apologized after a six-year-old leukaemia patient was wrongly given too much steroid medication for two months. (Anon in *Yorkshire Evening Post*, 27 March 2007)

The second type of story covered calls from various sources, such as Members of Parliament, individuals affected by patient safety failures, or organizations representing patients, to improve patient safety. The key source for these stories was typically the individual or organization making the call for improved safety, as in the following examples from *The Times* and the *Birmingham Post* respectively.

> Thousands of lives are being put at risk every year in the NHS because of the Government's failure to set up an effective system to monitor patient safety and prevent mistakes recurring, an influential cross-party committee said yesterday. (Lister in *The Times*, 6 July 2006)

> More needs to be done to cut hospital mistakes after figures revealed more than 40,000 medication errors in one year, the health regulator said yesterday. (Pinch in *Birmingham Post*, 12 August 2006)

The third category of coverage was of plans designed to improve patient safety, such as the World Health Organization's surgical safety checklist for use in operating theatres that the National Patient Safety Agency (NPSA) required NHS Trusts to implement by February 2010: 'Safety checklist to cut errors in operations for surgeons' (Smith in *The Daily Telegraph*, 15 January 2009). Another common area for safety improvement was in relation to medications:

> Drug safety watchdogs are preparing new guidance on prescribing, dispensing and administering anti-cancer and blood-thinning drugs after serious medication errors that have led to patients dying or being permanently harmed. (Meikle in *The Guardian*, 22 January 2004)

The source for this type of story was either the NHS or, since its establishment in 2002, the National Patient Safety Agency. Coverage of plans or innovations designed to improve patient safety usually referred to a serious incident from the past or to generic statistics on medical errors and accidents, as illustrated in the following extract:

> World-wide, an estimated 234 million operations are carried out a year, and about one million people die each year following major surgery (BBC, 25 June 2008)

Since our search located only one news story in the popular media that directly referenced a PSRP research study aimed at improving patient safety, yet found numerous stories covering serious or fatal patient incidents, offering strategies for improvement in their aftermath or making calls to improve patient safety from those affected by such incidents, we can suggest that patient safety tends to receive media coverage only when it is found to be lacking or deficient.

Rejecting 'Inaccuracy': Understanding News Media Coverage of Research

So how then are we to understand the selection of patient safety stories that receive coverage in the media? Moreover, what can we learn about why a programme of research specifically designed to improve safety for patients in the NHS and beyond was largely ignored within media coverage? Historically there has been a tendency for scientific and medical communities to criticize the media for their choice of scientific and medical stories and the style and manner that such coverage has taken (Nelkin 1996). Following this line of argument, coverage of patient safety 'failures', and the limited coverage of patient safety 'successes' or progress might be taken as further evidence to support the notion of a media that 'fails' to cover science, medicine or research in these areas, in an 'accurate' or educational manner. Such criticisms have however been convincingly critiqued in their own right by scholars examining the popular communication of scientific and medical research (Nelkin 1996, Gregory and Miller 1998, Seale 2002, Schudson 2003). These scholars draw attention to the fundamental assumptions underlying attacks on media 'accuracy'. Seale notes how '"inaccuracy" or misrepresentation in the media is perceived by critics to have a direct and potentially "damaging" effect of some kind' (2002: 51). A second and broader assumption on the part of such critics is that it is in some way the 'job', or obligation of the media to educate or inform 'the public' in a manner of which those who work in science and medicine would approve.

Nelkin identifies an 'enduring tension' between medicine and the media and suggests that 'perhaps the most important source of strain between scientists and journalists lies in their different views about the media's role' (1996: 1602). She outlines scientists' view of the media as documented by science communication scholar Jon Turney (1996):

> They view the press as a conduit or pipeline, responsible for transmitting science to the public in a way that can be easily understood. Scientists expect to control the flow of information to the public as they do within their own domain ... they assume that the purpose of science journalism is to convey a positive image; they see the media as a means of furthering scientific and medical goals. Most journalists, however, do not see themselves as trumpets for science. (Nelkin 1996: 1602)

In a similar vein, Gregory and Miller (1998) identify the propensity of scientists to engage in assertions regarding how the media 'should' be working. They argue 'high on scientists' agenda has been the question of accuracy – that is, the extent to which popularizations faithfully reproduce the facts of science ... this has served to perpetuate an image of popular media as misrepresenting science' (Gregory and Miller 1998: 107). These scholars identify the tendency on the part of scientific and medical researchers to assume that the role of the media is to provide a positive and accurate account of scientific and medical research that will inform and educate the public in line with a worldview similar to their own. Where journalists or media coverage fail to live up to such expectations, accusations of inaccuracy, misrepresentation or scaremongering often follow. A further criticism of media stories, particularly regarding coverage of scientific or medical research findings, is that that they are sensationalist, as a result of exaggeration, over-simplification or attempts to stimulate the emotions of their audience.

Despite their re-evaluation by sociologists, scientific and medical criticisms of media coverage are not without foundation. Multiple studies have demonstrated the media's preference for certain stories over others, and the use of narratives and metaphors to frame issues in particular ways. For example, Entwistle's (1995) study of research coverage in medical journals and newspapers found that:

> Journalists stressed that medically worthy information is not necessarily newsworthy. They said they were more likely to cover currently topical subjects, common and fatal diseases; rare but interesting or quirky diseases; those with a sexual connection; new or improved treatments; and controversial subject matter or results (1995: 3).

Entwistle also made a particularly interesting finding regarding the studies that did not receive coverage in the newspapers. She found that these studies 'did not involve high technology medicine and related more to social problems than biomedical problems, which are more commonly covered by the media' (1995: 3). A further study evidencing the types of stories favoured by the media is Bartlett et al.'s (2002) longitudinal study, which examined the selection by medical journal editors of research articles that would be included in a press release, and the subsequent selection of newsworthy stories by journalists. Bartlett's study found that although '"good" and "bad" news were equally likely to be press released, the newspapers tended to report the bad news' (2002: 83). They also found that 'randomized trials, which represent the gold standard for evaluation of medical interventions, were underreported in newspapers despite their being more likely to be included in press releases' (Bartlett et al. 2002: 83). This finding seems to have caused particular concern to the authors, who end their paper with a particularly neat example of normative theorizing (see Gregory and Miller 1998) in relation to the role of the press:

> We are concerned that many aspects of medical research are not well represented in newspapers ... newspapers have a role to play in health care – for example, by explaining the importance of evidence from randomized controlled trials, dispelling the misconceptions and confusion that surround the concepts of randomization and equipoise, and reporting both good and bad news and research that is relevant to international health (Bartlett et al. 2002: 84).

Both Entwistle's (1995) and Bartlett et al.'s (2002) studies examine and illustrate the selection of stories about medical research on the part of journalists or media organizations and find, somewhat unsurprisingly, that journalists choose to cover certain topics over others. Controversial, unusual or negative subjects received coverage whereas research that explored social aspects of health, randomized trials of medical interventions or studies with non-British authors were excluded altogether. These two studies differ however in terms of how they choose to interpret their findings: the extract above from Bartlett expresses 'concern' about misrepresentation on the part of the media, concluding with the expectation that the media 'should' report in a different way, should cover aspects of research that currently it does not, and should be educative for the reader. This extract is a good example of a call for the media to change itself, or to do a 'better' job. However, defining the coverage of science and medical stories as inaccurate or misrepresentative imposes a scientific criteria of accuracy on the media; this might be considered unfair as, quite clearly, the media does not belong to scientists. Entwistle (1995) follows an alternative line of interpretation and rather than lament how the media ought to work, she turns her attention to the realities and constraints of news production. This approach seeks to understand the media for what it is, rather than what it should be. Such approaches refrain from judging media outputs against scientifically defined criteria of accuracy, and instead understand these outputs as products of a particular culture which are designed to serve a certain purpose.

Similarly to Entwistle (1995), the work of scholars such as Nelkin (1996), and Gregory and Miller (1998) incorporates an understanding of the working realities of journalism to illustrate that accusations of media inaccuracy or misrepresentation on the part of scientists fail to acknowledge or accept the different cultures occupied by the scientist and the scientific or medical journalist. Tim Radford, former science editor of UK broadsheet newspaper *The Guardian*, sums up the key imperative of the print media quite simply: 'to tell stories ... the day the readers stop reading, they stop buying, and the newspaper dies' (2009: 152). With this simple but profoundly important imperative of media culture stated, he goes on:

> Even the science stories in newspapers are just that, stories. They are drawn from the world of science. They are told for serious purpose. But they are told so as to give pleasure. It is not our business to advance the public education in science, except by the way, and as a kind of happy accident. It is our business to be read (Radford 2009: 152).

While scientists and researchers may expect the media to transmit their work to the public in an accurate and educative way, journalists and news producers are expected to produce stories that are likely to be read or otherwise consumed by the public. Seale further elaborates on the imperative of media forms 'to be read': 'emotional engagement of audiences is the key task for news, advertising, fiction and other media forms. Media organizations are largely driven by the need to acquire, keep and expand their audiences' (2002: 40). To state what should perhaps be obvious, scientists and journalists occupy different cultures with unique objectives. The style of output that advances a scientist's career and perpetuates the institutions engaged in medical or scientific research is fundamentally different from that which will support a journalist and preserve the existence of the media organization for which they work. Stories that adhere to scientific standards of accuracy may not be those that attract or engage the reader. Appealing to the public is likely to require a style of reporting that differs greatly from the strictly educational or informative tone that might be favoured by scientists aiming to have their work understood and appreciated in nuanced detail. As Nelkin notes, the objective of media stories 'to be read' often entails the stripping away of features assuring the scientific imperative 'to be accurate': 'media constraints of time, brevity, and simplicity preclude the careful documentation, nuanced positions, and precautionary qualifications that scientists feel are necessary to present their work' (1996: 1601). She further notes that in the search for a human interest angle: 'journalists look for personal stories and individual cases, though this may distort research that has meaning only in a broader statistical context' (1996: 1601).

News Values and Coverage of Patient Safety Issues

Reconsidering the findings of our media review in light of the argument to approach media outputs as products of a particular culture, the core imperative of which is to engage the reader, it is possible to make some claims as to why patient safety failures received extensive coverage, whereas a programme of research designed to improve patient safety was largely ignored. A number of scholars (Nelkin 1996, Seale 2002) have reflected and elaborated on the concept of 'news values' as first defined by Galtung and Ruge (1973). 'News values' refer to certain characteristics or features of a story that make it 'newsworthy', and following the discussion above, newsworthiness is that which will get the audience engaged, and the story read. Galtung and Ruge's news values are summarized by Seale as follows:

> Negative, recent, close to home, compatible with dominant stereotypes, unambiguous, novel or unexpected, superlative … relevant to an audience's daily life experience, personalized, involving important people or sources, and containing certain kinds of hard facts such as places, numbers, names (2002: 39).

With these news values in mind, it is possible to see why stories about failures or deficiencies in patient safety have received considerable coverage. To reiterate, our media search located three broad categories of patient safety news story. Most common were those about serious incidents, followed by coverage of calls to improve safety, and coverage of plans to improve patient safety. Patient safety failures are indeed negative; they are by definition 'bad news' stories. Patient safety failure stories are unambiguous in that a tragic incident has occurred for which there is no justification, an innocent victim and a clear perpetrator in the form of the hospital or health setting involved. Furthermore, failures in patient safety have a novel and unexpected quality because they embody a neat yet dramatic irony; the system in which the audience places their faith as a source of healing and care can be shown instead as a source of grave personal risk. This irony also fulfils the value of relevance 'to an audience's life experience', since the vast majority of news media consumers are NHS patients and therefore cannot help but be drawn to an account of a tragic event involving the NHS. To this end, we found that personalization was common throughout media coverage. Patient safety stories about calls or plans to improve patient safety commonly contained references to past serious incidents at specified hospitals, and made use of statistics on medical error and accidents. Examples of such references can be found in news media stories reporting the introduction of the surgical safety checklist for use in operating theatres, as in the following example from *The Daily Telegraph*: 'in England and Wales, 129,419 incidents relating to surgical specialties were reported to the NPSA's Reporting and Learning System in 2007 with 217 deaths' (Smith 2009).

If we apply the above criteria to the PSRP research studies, and consider them in relation to academic research more generally, academic research can to an extent be seen to resist the characteristics or features deemed to make a story newsworthy. Patient safety failures are located in complex systems, far from the fault of identifiable individuals. Therefore patient safety research turns its attention to in-depth understanding of specific aspects of the deeply complex organization of the health service, how these function and how they may engender either risk or safety in the delivery of patient care. Such a focus is depersonalized and specific to aspects of health service design and organization that are far from familiar to the life experiences of a lay person. Furthermore, the research findings of the patient safety studies, as with all research studies, are careful, measured and qualified, rather than final or definitive. This feature is summed up by Gregory and Miller, who suggest that 'everything is moderated and qualified ... no claim can be too small' (1998: 110). Uncertainty is freely acknowledged, as symbolized by the eternal refrain that concludes research papers from many fields that 'more research is needed'. Given these qualifications and moderations, research provides neither good news nor bad news stories, but rather a series of careful, nuanced interpretations on the small scale. This is the very opposite of the superlative tendency found in media reports. Consider Radford's articulation in which he reflects on the features of research papers:

> I am ... confronted, when I open *Nature* or *Science* or the *Proceedings of the Royal Society*, by papers that consist of a series of unemotional statements, hedged with caveat and festooned with proviso, couched in deliberately passive sentences, and phrased in wilfully opaque language (2009: 147–148).

Newsworthiness requires stories to be relevant, unambiguous and clear-cut, whereas research studies present incremental findings referring to the complexity and uncertainty of the world. The absence of characteristics or features deemed 'newsworthy' could perhaps explain the virtual exclusion of PSRP research studies from the media as indicated by our media review. However, different forms of complex scientific, medical and social scientific research can and do receive media coverage every day. In this final section, it is the scientific press release, we will argue, that represents the key to this dislocation and is the fundamental reason why PSRP research received minimal news coverage.

Before Newsworthiness: the Role of the Press Release

As we have argued, criteria of newsworthiness play a major role in determining whether a research study receives media coverage. However, journalists must first become or be made aware of the research study in question before judgments as to its newsworthiness can be made. Indeed, it could be argued that a piece of research does not intrinsically possess or lack 'news value'. Rather this news value is determined and attributed by the producers of media outputs as and when they become aware of the study concerned. The primary means by which journalists become aware of scientific and medical research (and indeed of many other topical events) is the press release. As we have previously noted,

> Unless a story is actively presented to a journalist via a press release or direct contact, it is unlikely to feature on their radar. In particular, research that is published in journals that do not produce press releases is very unlikely to be picked up by the popular media (Dingwall et al. 2009: 41).

Journalists are expected to produce a high number of stories daily, which immediately limits the amount of time that they can dedicate to uncovering stories. Contrary to popular depictions of journalists engaging in investigative practices, the vast majority of science stories across all forms of UK news media are prompted by press releases, press briefings or direct communication between journalists and researchers. Few stories are produced by the journalist uncovering stories though sources and contacts, rather it might be said that the stories seek out the journalist: 'the vast majority of daily news comes from planned, intentional events, press releases, press conferences, and scheduled interviews' (Schudson 2003: 5–6). Science and health journalists receive regular press releases from all major health journals including the *Lancet*, the *British Medical Journal*, the *New England Journal of Medicine* and *Journal of the American Medical Association*. Press releases are also received from government bodies, health-based charities, health care Trusts and private health organizations. Other media outlets and the news agencies Reuters or Associated Press are further sources of stories. Dependent on budget, news media organizations may also receive some professional journals, likely to be a small number of the major publications such as *BMJ* or the *Lancet* (see Entwistle 1995). However, journalists are prevented by time constraints from seeking out research journals over and above those made available to them, and without a press release journalists are highly unlikely to be aware of a research study at all.

The search of university press release archives undertaken as part of our search for media coverage of the PSRP studies found that the vast majority of researchers and hosting institutions had not attempted to promote or promulgate the findings of their studies though the mass media. In contrast, the patient safety media stories we did find, which focused on failures or deficiencies, could be linked to a press release, briefing or public statement from individuals or organizations affected by, or with a professional interest in, the issue of patient safety. Furthermore, the primary investigator of the only PSRP study we found to have received media coverage, informed us that his institution had released a press release about the study (although we were unable to confirm this, since the press release archive on the Manchester University website does not provide access to releases more than three years old). The press release is a key link in the chain between research studies in specialist academic and professional publications and their translation into widespread coverage in the popular press. The press release not only makes the journalist aware of the study concerned, it also presents and summarizes the most newsworthy aspects of the research findings and packages them in a way that makes it easy for the time-pressured journalist to write a story. As Entwistle's exploration of research reporting in the newspapers states: 'media relations efforts can influence selection of stories by bringing information to journalists' attention, presenting it as newsworthy, and making a news article easier to write' (1995: 2).

Although putting a press release out in no way guarantees media coverage (there will always be competition from many other newsworthy items) it seems likely that had a greater number of PSRP studies been press released, more extensive media interest and media coverage may have followed. Press releases about the PSRP programme as a whole might also have led to increased awareness about the initiative on the part of specialist journalists. We were not able to collect data as to why so few PSRP research teams sought to engage with the media, as it fell beyond the remit of the study. However, there is a common consensus, supported by funders such as the Medical Research Council and Wellcome Trust, that it is worthwhile and beneficial for researchers to engage with, and publish their work in the popular media. It is argued that engaging with the media fulfils a responsibility to the taxpayer to inform them of the work being undertaken by taxpayer-funded researchers. Specific to patient safety research, it could be argued that because the vast majority of the lay public obtain information from the popular media, successes in research aimed at improving patient safety should be disseminated via the same outlets. Dissemination in this way also has the potential to reach professionals who might be involved in implementing best practice and informing them of recent developments and potential collaborators in the patient safety field.

This chapter has explored the paradox of patient safety in the media; namely that patient safety receives coverage primarily when found to be failing or deficient in some way, whereas positive patient safety stories, covering improvements or advances in patient safety, are largely absent. This was found to be the case in relation the Patient Safety Research Portfolio, our assessment of which found only a single identifiable news story in the UK news media. The chapter has reflected on the tensions that have at times characterized the relationship between those engaged in research and those tasked with writing news stories, and suggests that, rather than holding the media to a standard of accuracy imposed by a different professional world, scientists and researchers might be better advised to reconsider their expectations of the media and its outputs. In so doing there is great potential to work with the media as it is, rather than despair of it as it should be. Researchers who wish their work to receive popular coverage would be well advised to make things as easy as possible for journalists, who are under greater pressure to produce more stories in less time (Williams and Clifford 2009). As such, this chapter concludes with a potential strategy for engaging with the media, developed from the experience of one of the authors who is a science journalist with 15 years experience of broadcast and print media (TM).

Media Engagement Strategies for Patient Safety Researchers

Identifying and building relationships with the individuals responsible for particular kinds of stories is important. In the case of patient safety research, the medical or health correspondent is the logical choice. Producers of health programmes or social affairs editors may also be useful. Press releases cannot be guaranteed to reach the relevant reporter, so identifying the correct individuals who could be notified about a research study and potential stories that might be derived from it, is key.

A productive strategy for contacting a journalist is likely to be a short initial telephone call to check that they are the correct person to contact, and to ask how they would like to receive further information. Journalists do not have the time to read or respond to long emails or extensive documents. It is also pertinent to be sensitive about the time of day: a daily print journalist will have a copy deadline of around 16:00, and will not appreciate a phone call at 15:45.

- Because journalists are time pressured, stories will have a better chance of coverage if they are clearly explained, and have contributors ready to provide an interview and further information or images suitable for newspaper use. With the possible exception of news websites, media outlets are restricted in the number of stories they can cover because their column space or allocated airtime is limited. This results in strong competition for stories as journalists compete for space and airtime. A concise, clearly worded press release will help a journalist to persuade their editor to run with their story.

- Journalists look for stories that will chime with their audience, and certain stories will be deemed more relevant for certain audiences. Finding the human element to a story works well, as does linking up with patient interest groups; offering an interview with someone who has been campaigning for a change in practice brings human interest to the story and makes it easier for the journalist to sell it to their editor.

- With a topic such as patient safety, it is impossible to avoid bad news. Informing the journalist of a patient safety incident that the research study is aimed at preventing from happening again is likely to raise their interest.

- A big news story breaking during the day can knock all other stories either down, or completely off the schedule. Further, journalists may be under pressure to mould or reform their stories to the desires of the editor. A journalist may therefore promise to run with a story only for it not to appear at all, or to appear in a radically revised form. While disconcerting, the media-savvy researcher will accept these setbacks as a consequence of the media process.

- Awards of grant money are not commonly seen as newsworthy. However, there was potential for the PSRP to be a news story in its own right because the funding programme was aimed specifically at making encounters with the medical profession safer for patients. Making journalists aware of a new programme of research is an opportunity to let them know about the range of planned studies and to alert them to upcoming stories.

- At regular intervals the progress of a programme of research should be assessed to see if there is a suitable story for a press release. However, if a number of studies report within a short space of time it is recommended to highlight one or two rather than overwhelm the press with a flood of press releases.

- Each press release should have the potential to be a story, even if only a small one. Researchers should be cautious of making frivolous contact with journalists, as regular but useless press releases may be seen as 'crying wolf'.

- Research studies with negative or inconclusive results are less likely to be deemed worth reporting, but they can be bracketed as areas where the research has found that further work is needed. Under no circumstances should any attempt be made to conceal or ignore such studies, as an organization attempting to hide something from public scrutiny is always a good story for a journalist.

- Finally, the media regularly cannibalizes older stories, therefore the existence of stories within the cuttings database means that they are more likely to be followed up in the future, or used as sources for new and different stories.

References

Anon. 2007. Heartache for family over boy's leukaemia medicine blunder. *Yorkshire Evening Post*, 27 March.

Bartlett, C., Sterne, J. and Egger, M. 2002. What is newsworthy? Longitudinal study of the reporting of medical research in two British newspapers. *British Medical Journal*, 325, 81–84.

BBC. 2008. *Safety Checklist For Ops Launched*. Available from http://news.bbc.co.uk/go/pr/fr/-/1/hi/health/7472705.stm.

Department of Health. 2000. *An Organization with a Memory*. London: The Stationery Office.

Dingwall, R., Palmer, C., Rowley, E., Waring, J. and Murcott T. 2009. *Synthesis of the Outputs of Research Commissioned Under the Patient Safety Research Portfolio*. Birmingham: PSRP.

Entwistle, V. 1995. Reporting research in medical journals and newspapers. *British Medical Journal*, 310, 920–923. Available at http://www.bmj.com/content/310/6984/920.full.

Galtung, J. and Ruge, M. 1973. Structuring and selecting news, in *The Manufacture of News*, edited by S. Cohen and J. Young. London: Constable and Co, pp. 62–72.

Gregory, J. and Miller, S. 1998. *Science in Public: Communication, Culture and Credibility*. New York: Basic Books.

Healthcare Commission. 2009. *Investigation into Mid-Staffordshire NHS Foundation Trust* (Commission for Healthcare Audit and Inspection). London: Healthcare Commission.

Lilford, R., Foster, J., Stoddart, S. and Maillard, N. 2005. *PSRP Standard Operating Procedures Summary*. PSRP internal document.

Lister, S. 2006. NHS 'not learning from errors'. *The Times*, 6 July, 29.

Meikle, J. 2004. New rules planned to cut drugs errors. *The Guardian*, 22 January, 7.

Millenson, L. 2002. Pushing the profession: how the news media turned patient safety into a priority. *Quality and Safety in Healthcare*, 11, 57–63.

Nelkin, D. 1996. An uneasy relationship: the tensions between medicine and the media. *Lancet*, 347(9015), 1600–03. Available at http://www.sciencedirect.com/science?_ob=MImg&_imagekey=B6T1B-4B8JM79-1WB-1&_cdi=4886&_user=5939061&_pii=S0140673696910818&_origin=search&_coverDate=06%2F08%2F1996&_sk=996520984&view=c&wchp=dGLbVlW-zSkzk&md5=06b5ed26a70820f4c6982a90dae616ef&ie=/sdarticle.pdf.

Pinch, E. 2006. Hospitals shamed on medicine errors. *Birmingham Post*, 12 August, 2.

Radford, T. 2009. A workbench view of science communication and metaphor in *Communicating Biological Sciences: Ethical and Metaphorical Dimensions*, edited by B. Nerlich, R. Elliott and B. Larson. Farnham: Ashgate, pp. 145–52.

Sandars, J. and Esmail, A. 2001. *Threats to Patient Safety in Primary Care: a Review of the Research into the Frequency and Nature of Error in Primary Care*. Birmingham: PSRP.

Schudson, M. 2003. *The Sociology of News*. New York: W.W Norton and Company.

Seale, C. 2002. *Media and Health*. London: Sage.

Smith, R. 2009. Safety checklist to cut errors in operations for surgeons. *The Daily Telegraph*, 15 January, 8.

Stebbing, C. and Kaushal, R. 2006. Pediatric medication safety and the media: what does the public see? *Pediatrics*, 117, 1907–14.

Turney, J. 1996. Public understanding of science. *Lancet*, 347, 1087–90.

Williams, A. and Clifford, S. 2009. *Mapping the Field: Specialist Science News Journalism in the UK National Media*. Cardiff: Cardiff University, The Risk, Science and the Media Research Group.

Wright, O. 2003. GPs will own up to errors in 'near miss' log. *The Times*, 21 May, 4.

Chapter 2

Broadening the Patient Safety Movement: Listening, Involving and Learning from Patients and the Public

Josephine Ocloo

In patient safety, it is increasingly being recognized that in developing a patient safety culture, there has been little discussion about what can be learned from the perspectives of patients and the public, and particularly those affected by patient safety incidents. This chapter examines some of the key drivers for involvement more generally in health care and then looks more specifically at the emergence of a patient and public involvement (PPI) agenda in patient safety. A key objective is to look at evidence of progress in developing strategies for involvement in patient safety in the light of the considerable patient safety movement that has developed over the last ten years in health care.

Whilst there is a wealth of literature on the involvement of individual patients in their own disease-specific treatment, care and decision-making, *involvement* in patient safety is a narrower and comparatively under-researched area. Peat and colleagues (2010) have identified three broad areas by which patients' actions might contribute to their safety. These relate to initiatives to ensure the safety of a patient's treatment (through informing the patient about their management plan or monitoring them to ensure safe delivery of treatment) or involvement initiatives connected to systems improvement in addressing how problems with risks are identified and improved. In exploring the involvement literature on patient safety, consideration is given to looking at current ways of conceptualizing and researching the evidence to see what lessons can be learned in the context of a much wider discourse on user involvement that has emerged in other parts of the public sector. This discourse suggests that the emergence of user involvement raises important questions about power inequities in service provision, which have also strongly challenged a biomedical model of health and illness in treatment and decision-making. This is considered to have implications for further developing an involvement agenda in patient safety that goes beyond paternalism to patient empowerment.

Drivers for Involvement in Health

It is within the context of the development of user involvement in broader welfare and public services that the UK's policy and legislative imperative for user participation emerged in health care. The establishment of the Community Health Councils in 1973 marked a turning point in which the rhetoric of user involvement became a central component of NHS policy. Baggott (2005) argues the 'new managerialist' conservative reforms of the 1980s and 1990s emphasized the need to engage with service users, but mainly resulted from management imperatives to demonstrate support for specific plans and policies. Significant policy developments in the 1990s saw the implementation of the NHS and Community Care Act 1990, which was the first piece of UK legislation to formally establish a requirement for user involvement in service planning. Further policy developments included the Patient's Charter (Department of Health 1991) and plans set out in *Local Voices* (NHS Management Executive 1992), which stressed the need to make services more responsive to patients needs (Tait and Lester 2005, Tritter and Lester 2007). However, despite these initiatives, an influential report from the Institute for Public Policy Research identified a democratic deficit in health that has acted to exclude the participation of citizens in the planning of public services and decision-making. This paved the way for a much more radical debate about how to achieve greater public participation and citizen engagement in health processes (Cooper et al. 1995).

The late 1990s eventually saw a distinct shift in the language of user involvement in health care, with the emergence of a strong policy and later in 2001, a legal imperative, which emphasized the importance of patient and public involvement as part of New Labour's NHS modernization agenda. In health care practice, this commitment to user involvement came much later than in other parts of the public sector.

A key emphasis driving policy developments has been to stress the importance of participation as an important way of improving the performance of health care services (Baggott 2005). Rutter and colleagues (2004) have suggested that the participation of service users can improve the quality of services, clarify what patients want and enhance democratic principles. The development of this agenda was given greater momentum by the evidence from serious clinical and service failings in health care, highlighted in the UK by high-profile inquiries (for example, children's heart surgery in Bristol, Alder Hey, Royal Liverpool Children's Inquiry 2001, which examined the retention of patients' organs without consent, and the Shipman Inquiry 2001–2005, which looked into the murders of large numbers of patients by the GP Harold Shipman). These inquiries highlighted the importance of developing safety cultures that dealt both with the prevention of harm to patients, as well as reinforced demands from the public for greater accountability from health care services and regulatory bodies (Davies and Shields 1999, Irvine 2004). The Bristol Royal Infirmary Inquiry Report was particularly important in stressing the need for PPI to be treated as a central feature in building a safety culture, both as a way to prevent the occurrence of errors and ameliorate the effects of harm to patients (Bristol Royal Infirmary Inquiry 2001).

This thinking has since led to a bewildering range of policy initiatives on involvement in health care (Department of Health 1999, 2000, 2003a, 2006). These have emphasized the benefits of PPI in improving the quality of individual care and in making changes to improve the performance of wider systems and services. More recent attempts to develop and embed PPI across NHS services have seen *World Class Commissioning* (Department of Health 2007), Lord Darzi's *High Quality Care For All: NHS Next Stage Review* (Department of Health 2008a) and the *NHS Constitution* (Department of Health 2010a): all reflect the shift of involvement to the forefront of the policy agenda and to recognize this as one of the key challenges to be addressed by NHS organizations. Current requirements to involve patients in their care and treatment are reflected in registration requirements for all NHS Trusts (Care Quality Commission 2009). The NHS Act (s242 (1B) 2006) also places a legal duty on NHS organizations to make arrangements to involve and consult with patients and the public on the planning and provision of services and in the development of proposals for change. Yet despite this considerable momentum to involve patients and the public in health care over the last ten years, there is still little evidence that involvement is a mainstream activity that sits alongside other policy and performance requirements in the NHS (Department of Health 2008b, Healthcare Commission 2009, Parsons et al. 2010).

The Development of Patient and Public Involvement in Patient Safety

In patient safety, a number of documents have set out clear expectations for NHS Trusts to develop PPI in patient safety and more recently at board level (National Leadership Council 2010). The document *Clinical governance in the new NHS* sets out clear expectations for NHS Trusts to develop PPI as an integral part of this work (NHS Executive 1999). *Safety first* (Department of Health 2006) outlines a national approach to developing patient safety in the NHS, and recommends that patients and carers are enabled to play an integral part in all initiatives to introduce a patient safety culture change within the NHS. Part of this approach included the establishment of a national network of patient champions to work in partnership with NHS organizations, as well as requiring health care organizations to implement local initiatives to promote greater openness with patients and their families when things went wrong with their health care. In developing the considerable reforms to professional regulation post the Shipman reports (2001–2005), *Tackling concerns locally – report of the clinical governance subgroup*, strongly highlights the importance of patient, public and carer involvement as central to the delivery of high-quality health care. The report highlights involvement as providing an important 'early warning' alongside other indicators, 'that the conduct or performance of a health care professional is slipping below acceptable standards' (Department of Health 2009: 3).

Despite these recommendations, Vincent and Coulter have noted that what is most remarkable about the multifaceted nature of the patient safety movement is 'the lack of attention paid to the patient' (Vincent and Coulter 2002: 76). Their research highlights that there are actually a number of areas in practice where patients can contribute to the safety of their care. For example, in helping to reach an accurate diagnosis, choosing an appropriate treatment, management strategy or safe provider, ensuring treatment is properly adhered to and monitored, and identifying adverse events and side effects and acting upon them.

Coulter and Ellins (2006) have reinforced this evidence in their systematic review of the patient safety literature. They note that whilst research in this area is still in its infancy, key findings show that patients want greater openness and honesty from health professionals when affected by patient safety incidents (PSIs). Patients were also thought to have the most potential in ensuring the safety of their care and to prevent the occurrence of errors in key areas such as making informed choices about providers, helping to reach an accurate diagnosis, sharing decisions about treatment and procedures, contributing to safe medication use, participating in infection control initiatives, checking the accuracy of medical records, observing and checking care processes, identifying and reporting treatment complications and adverse events, practising effective self-management, including treatment monitoring and shaping the design and improvement of services (Coulter and Ellins 2006). To develop this agenda further, they recommend the development of innovative strategies to support patients and health professionals to work in partnership, while arguing that these would 'need to be subjected to formal evaluation so that best practice could be identified and applied across settings' (Coulter and Ellins 2006: 172).

Despite these opportunities for involvement, in areas such as clinical governance in NHS Trusts there appears to be little evidence of successful strategies to promote patient and public involvement (Pickard et al. 2002). The National Audit Office reports (2003, 2007) covering both acute and primary care found that PPI remained one of the least well-developed components of clinical governance arrangements. Some evidence of good practice is provided by Fleming-Caroll and colleagues (2006) study, which looked at families as partners in a patient safety committee in a hospital environment focused on caring for acute and chronically ill children. This work was guided by principles of patient- and family-centred care, which respected and was responsive to individual patient preferences, needs and values in guiding clinical decisions, in conjunction with the entire family. The authors concluded that 'a task-oriented partnership between families and health care workers has proven to be a productive model for advancing paediatric patient safety' (Fleming-Caroll et al. 2006: 96).

More generally, however, what is clear from recent evidence emerging from inquiry reports into clinical failings in the NHS (Colin-Thomé 2009, Mid Staffordshire NHS Foundation Trust Inquiry 2010), is that there has been a distinct lack of progress in involving patients and the public in patient safety. Given this context, the publication of the White Paper 'Equity and excellence: liberating the

NHS' (Department of Health 2010b), with its strong rhetorical stance on PPI, provides an important opportunity to consider how involvement in the patient safety agenda can be further developed.

Peat and colleagues (2010) argue that a key priority now in developing the PPI agenda in patient safety is to explore 'how and how well existing and future interventions might support patients' contributions to patient safety in different contexts' (Peat et al. 2010: 24). In exploring this issue further, this chapter poses a more fundamental question about the way in which the whole debate on involvement in patient safety has been conceptualized. What is raised is the issue of the absence of a more critical discourse around involvement, which leads to questions about values, the contested nature of involvement and the way in which issues of power, conflict and the empowerment of patients and the public have been largely ignored in the construction of a patient safety movement over the last decade. Addressing these issues is seen as fundamental if more progress is to be made regarding PPI in patient safety.

Conceptualizing the Debate on Involvement

More broadly in patient safety, mainstream orthodoxy on developing a patient safety culture (Perrow 1984, Reason 1997) has concentrated on highlighting the role of systems and their design in causing error, rather than error occurring in organizations through the unsafe and individual acts of employees. Central to this thinking has been the notion of creating a non-punitive reporting environment that is just and fair to health professionals and which allows them to feel safe enough to report PSIs free from the threat of punishment and litigation (Reason 1997, Bristol Royal Infirmary Inquiry 2001). These ideas have assumed a dominant position in the approach to addressing patient safety internationally (Kohn et al. 1999, WHO 2005).

This situation is now being increasingly challenged, especially by those affected by PSIs, who have sought to open up a wider debate about medical harm and the construction of patient safety reforms, both nationally (Ocloo 2008) and internationally (WHO 2007, Newell et al. 2010). What is particularly noticeable about these perspectives is the way in which they have highlighted issues to do with the power of the medical profession and the failure of wider systems to deliver accountability when harm occurs to patients (Allsop et al. 2004, Fallowfield 2010, Ocloo 2010). This thinking on accountability, tied to the need to develop a 'just' organizational culture, has been far less recognized in initiatives to promote a safety culture in health care (Ocloo 2010). This is despite the recognition that governance and accountability are central to the performance of health care systems (WHO 2008). This situation raises difficult questions about developing a systems approach in patient safety that addresses the need for a non-punitive culture, whilst also delivering appropriate systems of justice and accountability that are fair to patients.

Broadening the patient safety discourse to include alternative perspectives from patients and the public is seen as important in a context where evidence-based medicine and the randomized clinical trial are viewed as 'the new gold standards in the health care field' (Timmermans and Berg 2003: 27). This backdrop has seen Leape and colleagues (2002) highlight the need to identify wider forms of knowledge and practice as part of developing a systems approach to patient safety than those produced through traditional biomedical research. Sharpe and Faden, taking the patients' perspective, have argued that the process of defining medical harm is not value free, but tends 'to reflect a narrowly clinical interpretation of harm that excludes non-clinical or non-disease-specific outcomes that the patient may consider harmful' (2001: 116). Consequently, there is a need for a broader knowledge framework for the evaluation of medical harm and the imposition of risk that is based upon a more patient-centred ethos (Sharpe and Faden 2001).

From a broader social science perspective, the limitations of a biomedical approach have long been criticized by medical sociologists for focusing primarily on the individual body as the primary unit of analysis when explaining disease, rather than the socially constructed nature of health and illness (Bury 1986, Nettleton 1995). Writing about medicalization in the USA, Conrad (2005) has strongly suggested that there is a need for sociologists to adopt a much wider political and economic perspective when looking at processes that cause considerable harm to patients. Whilst doctors are still seen as the gatekeepers in terms of access to many drugs, he argues that it is the pharmaceutical companies that have now become the major drivers in medicalization, in aggressively promoting their products to doctors and directly to the public (Conrad and Leiter 2004, Conrad 2005). Summerton and Berner also raise issues when looking at risk, about the need to understand 'everyday interactive practices' (Summerton and Berner 2003: 19) through which different actors construct safety. From this viewpoint they argue:

> Risks are collective – but often contested – outcomes that emerge in situated experiences and socially embedded interactions. An important task is thus to analyze the interpretations and meanings that actors ascribe to both risk phenomena and the interactions through which these evolve (Summerton and Berner, 2003: 19).

Understanding the experiences of harmed patients is therefore considered to provide a unique alternative standpoint to the dominant viewpoint of the medical profession in highlighting broader social processes to do with power and control that construct harm and go well beyond the original patient safety incident. For example in 2009, the Health Select Committee Report into patient safety highlighted various systemic processes that failed to ensure that when a patient was harmed they (and their families/carers) received a full and open explanation; apology and an undertaking that all necessary steps would be taken to avoid the same harm coming to another patient in the future (House of Commons 2009).

They concluded that whilst the NHS had made some progress in this respect, too often there was still a lack of frankness on all these accounts (House of Commons 2009).

Key systems identified as failing patients in addressing their concerns were complaints procedures, coroner's inquiries and lack of independent support from NHS Patient Advice and Liaison Services. Their strongest criticism was aimed at the failure of the then Labour government to implement the NHS Redress Scheme 2006 (as an alternative to litigation on claims up to £15,000 through the courts), despite passing the necessary legislation. This situation was viewed as hindering the development of a safety culture, which could not be developed in the context of powerful competing interests between openness and medico–legal concerns (House of Commons 2009).

In analysing the experiences of harmed patients in the aftermath of a PSI, Vincent (2006) has long highlighted the further trauma caused to these patients when health professionals fail to take their complaints seriously and label individuals negatively after an adverse incident has occurred. In providing some explanation for the failure to deal with harmed patients' concerns, sociologists such as Annandale (1989) and Mulcahy (2000) have pointed to the negative stereotyping of patients who complain or take legal action as a way of deflecting blame away from the medical profession. These experiences raise important questions about power inequities and conflict that have been largely ignored in patient safety (Antonsen 2009). These issues have been well documented in other parts of health care, in looking at the links between medicine and the way it is mediated by social forces of power and control, which in turn have shaped medical knowledge and practice (Illich 1974, Taussig 1980, Wright and Treacher 1982, Bury 1986).

These critiques are therefore seen as having considerable relevance in developing an involvement agenda in patient safety. This more critical discourse has been central to the development of user involvement more broadly in other parts of the public sector.

With respect to this agenda, Cowden and Singh (2007) point to the late 1970s and throughout the 1980s as a particularly significant period in Britain, which saw a series of campaigns by disenfranchised groups and communities (Black, anti-racist, feminist, lesbian and gay and disability rights movements) take place around welfare services. In health care, this saw a number of health social movements (for example, women's groups challenging the medicalization of childbirth, disability and mental health groups rejecting a medical model as a source of oppression) act as an important political force in achieving broader social change (Brown and Zavestoski 2004). Health Social Movements (HSMs) can be seen as providing 'collective challenges to medical policy and politics, belief systems, research and practice that include an array of formal and informal organizations, supporters, networks of co-operation and media' (Brown and Zavestoski 2004: 52). In health care, these types of groups were vocal in challenging a wide range of oppressive behaviour and discrimination that has echoed campaigns in many other parts of the public services.

Connected to these challenges from user groups and social movements, related sociological arguments emerged. These criticized the limitations of a biomedical model of health and illness (Friedson 1970, Oakley 1976, Rogers and Pilgrim 1991) and challenged the nature of the more traditional and paternalistic doctor–patient relationships defined by sociologists such as Parsons (1951). This led to calls for new types of medical relationships in which the individual patient was more active (Gabe et al. 2005) and empowered (Freidson 1970) and which embraced more informed and shared models of treatment and decision-making (Charles et al. 1999, Rutter at al. 2004).

Other arguments focused on the way in which some groups experienced poorer and unequal access to health care (Townsend et al. 1988, Acheson 1998). Sociologists also highlighted concerns about the very nature and disabling effects of the professions and their role in the provision of health care iatrogenesis (Illich 1974, Illich et al. 1977, Schon 1983). These issues emerged alongside wider concerns in health to do with rising costs, litigation, the influence of the pharmaceutical industry and growing protest from patient groups (Blane 1991). These problems provided the basis for measures aimed at curbing the autonomy of the medical professions and addressing the traditional imbalance of power between doctors and patients (Freidson 1970, Blane 1991).

The emergence of an involvement agenda in patient safety and particularly challenges from harmed patients can therefore be seen as part of a new social movement in health care, which forms part of a much bigger discourse on involvement in health since the 1970s. This discourse has sought to challenge the dominance of a medical model and highlighted the importance of recognizing lay perspectives in defining health and illness. Campaigns by harmed patients, for example, Bristol 2001, Alder Hey 2001, Shipman 2001–2005, Mid-Staffordshire 2010, have been at the forefront of demands for change in patient safety, and their struggles have acted as a catalyst for a major shift in thinking in this area. This has stressed the importance of PPI both as a way of delivering safer care and improving the performance of health services, through a shift away from paternalism (Bristol Royal Infirmary Inquiry 2001, Donaldson 2008) to patient empowerment (Colin-Thomé 2009) and partnership (Vincent and Coulter 2002, Coulter and Ellins 2006). Developing a partnership approach in patient safety therefore reflects a broader shift in health care that recognizes the importance of placing patients and the public at the very centre of their care and decision-making (Department of Health 2010a). What is lacking with this agenda is an understanding of different ways in which patients and the public can be empowered to participate.

Empowering Practice in Health and Social Care

To date what appears to be lacking in discussions about empowerment and involvement in patient safety is recognition of the contested nature of involvement. This contested agenda raises issues about tackling power inequities, abuse and exclusion in the provision of services that have been well documented more broadly in health and social care. This has seen the emergence of a range of theories aimed at empowering service users who have challenged the nature of oppressive and discriminatory service provision (Beresford 2003). This situation sits in contrast to the largely atheoretical nature of much of the literature on PPI in patient safety (Peat et al. 2010). Theorizing involvement practice in patient safety is therefore considered a necessary stage in developing new approaches to involvement based upon patient empowerment and partnership.

A range of ideas about empowering service users currently exists in health and social care and have been instrumental in highlighting issues of power and conflict in organizational contexts that might be useful in contributing to a more structured approach to guide and evaluate involvement in patient safety. In exploring concepts of empowerment, Starkey (2003) argues that the term is contested and has its roots in many different traditions and movements (for example the civil rights, anti-racist, women's and disability movements, mutual aid etc.). She concludes that 'the liberational model of empowerment, focused upon people's lives and roles within society, is likely to be more relevant to people than consumerist definitions narrowly focused on having a voice within services' (Starkey 2003: 273). In looking at a consumerist approach to empowerment in health, she locates this approach in the Conservative party policy of the 1980s and 1990s, reflected in legislation such as the NHS and Community Care Act 1990, and the NHS Plan (Department of Health 2000). In the latter document, she argues, the empowerment of patients is seen to be transmitted through 'information provision and redress' (Starkey 2003: 276). A consumerist model of empowerment is therefore seen as 'defined by service providers and policy makers, and has a narrow, individualized focus on people's ability to make choices within predetermined service systems' (McLean, 1995 cited in Starkey 2003: 277). In contrast, a liberational model has been defined as:

> A process of personal growth and development which enables people not only to assert their personal needs and to influence the way in which they are met, but also to participate as citizens within a community ... empowerment implies that processes of social and civic life should be designed to support and enable the participation of those who have previously been excluded from them. This means that change has to take place within social systems as well as within individuals and within services. Barnes (1997: 71) cited in Starkey (2003: 277)

Braye (2000) points out that whilst these models of participation appear conceptually opposed, in practice they frequently operate alongside each other.

In social work and social care, the development of Anti-Oppressive Practice (AOP) has brought together different strands of thinking and is based upon the premise 'that society is unequal and that the problems faced by service users have a personal, cultural and structural dimension' (Dalrymple and Burke 2006: 49). Challenging oppressive practice is seen as the driving force of AOP (Adams et al. 1998), alongside the empowerment of individuals and communities.

Opening up a values discourse has been central to this thinking, which recognizes the role that values play in shaping organizational cultures which are never value free. Braye and Preston-Shoot (1995) have argued that in the context of social care provision, real change will require a number of key actions. At the heart of this is the need to reappraise the traditional balance of power between users and professionals, to take account of what users want rather than imposing oppressive and non-negotiated solutions upon them. A key requirement for practitioners from this approach will be the need to engage with users and their networks in ways that do not stereotype through age, disability or mental health, nor oppress people through their race, sex, sexuality or class status. This will require practitioners to challenge experienced oppression and inequities through individually focused goals, as well as at a structural level (Braye and Preston-Shoot 1995). Addressing this context has led Beresford (2000) to argue that in this respect, the professions of social work and social care are more advanced in the area of promoting user involvement than other related disciplines, even though these professions still have a long way to go in addressing oppressive and discriminatory practice.

This raises questions about the need for a more theoretically driven approach to developing PPI in patient safety. This needs to address how issues to do with power imbalances and inequities can be tackled between health care professionals and patients and how patients and the public can best be empowered to be involved.

Patient and Public Involvement in Patient Safety as Empowerment

The development of an empowerment agenda to drive patient and public involvement in patient safety was seen as a central component of the Bristol Royal Infirmary Inquiry Report. This report viewed greater PPI as the only way to move beyond a culture of continuing secrecy, anonymity and paternalism, to create a better-quality health service, giving patients and the public a much greater degree of ownership over their own health care and in decision-making processes, based upon patient empowerment (Bristol Royal Infirmary Inquiry 2001). A key challenge was seen as how to embed key principles of PPI in the NHS, and how to devise mechanisms to ensure these principles became a reality and went beyond tokenism in empowering patients. Post-Bristol, Kennedy (2003) – who chaired the inquiry – expanded upon his views on empowerment to argue that in the provision of health care, patients and doctors were both experts in their own fields and so should work in partnership together.

Almost ten years after Bristol, the Colin-Thomé Report (2009) on the failings at Mid Staffordshire NHS Trust has highlighted continuing issues about the need to empower patients and the public in their care and health service delivery. With respect to individual care, information, choice and the need for patients to be 'seen as equal partners in their own care' described as 'the meeting of two experts when a patient meets their clinician', is seen as vitally important (Colin-Thomé 2009: 18). More broadly, the report called for patients and the public to be provided with and made more aware of methods to support their engagement, particularly when and where they have concerns. This greater level of involvement included being able to hold organizations with a role in monitoring and commissioning services to account for ensuring patients and the public were involved in the 'design, delivery and quality assurance of health and care services' (Colin-Thomé 2009: 18).

Whilst there have been a number of attempts post-Bristol to facilitate greater PPI in health care and related to patient safety, more work clearly needs to be done in this area. In order to strengthen involvement in decision-making in the NHS, Section 11 of the Health and Social Care Act 2001 (now S242 of the consolidated NHS Act 2006) strengthened obligations to implement PPI in health care. The aim of the new duty was to introduce practice in the NHS that would reinforce accountability to local communities and create services more responsive to patients as well as encourage NHS trusts to build upon previous work in this area (Department of Health 2003a). In order to facilitate these goals a number of new mechanisms and bodies were set up by the UK government. These included the Commission for Patient and Public Involvement in Health (CPPIH). This was an independent body established to ensure that the voice of both the wider public and patients were heard on health matters, primarily through the setting up of Patient and Public Involvement Forums (PPIFs) attached to all NHS Trusts. Other new bodies set up at the same time were the Patient Advice and Liaison Services (PALS) within hospital Trusts to handle and resolve patient concerns and provide advice and information; the Independent Complaints and Advocacy Service (ICAS) was established to provide support to patients in England who had formal complaints against the NHS, and the Overview and Scrutiny committees (OSCs), which was made up of locally elected councillors with the power to scrutinize and improve health services and reduce health inequalities in local communities.

However, despite considerable criticism from a range of sources (Warwick 2006, Dyer 2007), both CPPIH and the PPIFs were abolished by the Local Government and Public Involvement in Health Act (2007). To replace these forums, the Act set up alternative bodies called Local Involvement Networks (LINks), to enable individuals to influence or change the way local NHS and social care services are delivered (Department of Health 2008c). The White Paper, '*Equity and excellence: liberating the NHS*' (Department of Health 2010b) has now set out proposals to abolish the LINks and to replace them with Local Health Watch organizations. The aim is to enable these bodies at a local level to strengthen the collective voice of patients in commissioning services and through promoting choice and complaints advocacy and to act as a source of intelligence for national healthwatch in being able to report concerns about providers and propose investigations.

Given the considerable changes that have taken place with bodies set up to promote PPI since the abolition of the CHC's and concerns about the effectiveness of these arrangements (Hogg 2007, Department of Health 2009), how these bodies are structured to enable them to empower patients and communities will be crucial. Current evidence from the National Association of LINks Members (NALM) suggests that there are strong concerns about how these bodies will be set up to ensure that they are effective. These relate to the need for them to have appropriate governance structures, independence in raising concerns and the need to be given sufficient funding (National Association of LINk Members 2011).

In the area of clinical governance the Department of Health (2009: 23–24) has recommended three key principles to inform action on developing PPI:

1. Health care organizations and their boards should seek to actively encourage lay input.
2. Health care organizations should define and promote opportunities for lay involvement.
3. Organizations need to identify existing barriers that exclude patient and lay involvement and establish what support is required to enable it to happen.

It is unclear how these principles are being put into practice, what factors support or hinder involvement processes and how barriers to involvement might be addressed. Research in this area by Peat and colleagues (2010) suggests that patient representatives in patient safety improvement are generally expected to operate within existing systems, which can constrain attempts to bring a consumer perspective to the design and improvement of services.

Given this context, empowerment strategies taken from health and social care could be used to inform and develop thinking on how to develop the involvement agenda further in patient safety. Braye and Preston-Shoot argue that as 'long as partnership and empowerment remain undefined in legislation, differing interpretations are possible' (1995: 102). They argue that partnership can mean 'anything from token consultation to a total devolution of power and control' (1995: 102), whilst similar confusions about empowerment fail to differentiate between 'the rights, choices and control demanded by the self-advocacy movement and the mechanisms of consumerism prescribed in policy guidance' (1995: 102). Warren argues genuine empowerment ultimately 'calls for a shift in the balance of power' (2007: 62). This will require a commitment from individual practitioners 'to a set of values and ethical principles that treat people as equals and promotes the social inclusion of all' (Warren 2007: 63), but is also dependant upon a strong organizational commitment to the values and principles of involvement.

Changing the balance of power in patient safety will require action in a number of areas to identify issues to do with power inequities between patients, the public and health professionals, and how these can be addressed. Silbey has argued that new research in this area should explore:

> Those features of complex systems that are elided in the talk of safety culture: normative heterogeneity and cultural conflict, competing sets of interests within organizations, and inequalities in power and authority. Silbey (2009: 343)

At the collective strategic level, one area that could be developed in order to build a partnership approach to patient safety is the work of the Patients for Patient Safety (PfPS) Champions, who are part of the World Health Organization World Alliance for Patient Safety (WHO 2007, Newell et al. 2010). In England, champions have been involved mainly at a regional level in clinical governance in Patient Safety Action Teams (PSATs), supported by the National Patient Safety Association (NPSA). However, experiences have been varied and as Anderson (2010) notes, 'a patient safety champion in every trust and routine involvement of patients in patient safety work, may be some way off yet' (Anderson 2010: 15). In places such as Canada, champions have been invited to sit on patient safety advisory committees at a regional and local level and have become involved with national safety initiatives. However, Burns makes the point 'that much work is still needed. Patients and families face challenges, the most critical being the need to convince more health care organizations and service providers to engage patients and families in every aspect of patient safety initiatives' (Burns 2008: 100).

In order to further develop the work of the champions, a strategic review of their work to assess impact has recognized the need to identify more ways of supporting these individuals (WHO 2010). This objective faces an additional obstacle in the UK with the abolition of the NPSA (Department of Health 2010c). Some ways to build upon this work at a local level would be for health organizations to collaborate with voluntary groups and bodies such as HealthWatch to identify opportunities for involvement in patient safety activities at the individual and collective level in their organizations. In order to support this work organizations would need to clearly identify what factors and barriers hinder involvement, what action is needed to address this and what support is needed for staff and lay members (particularly from disadvantaged or under-represented groups) to facilitate the involvement process.

The involvement literature on patient safety also outlines other areas at the individual level where patients and the public could be empowered to be involved. Coulter and Ellins argue, 'particular attention should be paid to improving means of communicating with and listening to patients on matters of safety, and enhancing the availability and quality of safety information for patients and the public' (2006: 143). Various writers (Vincent et al. 1998, Coulter and Ellins 2006, Davis et al. 2007) have noted that the extent to which individual patients can contribute to safety improvement will depend on key factors. For example, individual patient characteristics, complexity and seriousness of illness, perceived vulnerability to harm, language and communication, health care professionals knowledge, beliefs and status and openness to involvement and the ability to challenge health care professionals.

Peat and colleagues (2010) found that safety interventions that were most successful required patients and their representatives to be well-informed and knowledgeable. This capacity was found to vary between individuals and to be significantly affected by educational level, income, cognitive skills and cultural differences, which might affect patients' health beliefs and ability to utilize health services (Peat et al. 2010).

These factors suggest that health inequities (see Marmott Review 2010) must be taken into account when thinking about involvement strategies. When thinking about patient safety, evidence shows that some groups have long received poorer and more unequal access to health care services that has considerable implications for them in receiving safe care. For example The Disability Rights Commission (2006) has highlighted the considerable discrimination faced by people with mental health problems and/or learning disabilities using primary care services in England and Wales. These groups were found to be less likely to receive important evidence-based treatments and health checks compared to others with the same condition, but without a learning disability or mental health problem. The Kings Fund (2006) and London Health Observatory (2005) have also highlighted a number of key issues on health inequalities and access affecting Black and minority ethnic communities. This picture of inequality in health care has also been reinforced more recently by the Parliamentary and Health Service Ombudsman, who highlighted 'a picture of NHS provision that is failing to respond to the needs of older people with care and compassion and to provide even the most basic standards of care' (2011: foreword).

Addressing these concerns will require the need to take a differentiated approach to involvement that targets specific patient groups' and identifies their needs, tackles discrimination and health inequities and empowers patients to challenge poor and unsafe practice and to raise their concerns. With the latter point, this is particularly required in a context where patient dissatisfaction with how their complaints have been handled has been well documented in health over many years (Department of Health 2003b, National Audit Office 2008).

Conclusion

This chapter has argued that despite the much-publicized discourse in patient safety about achieving patient and public involvement over the last ten years, there has still been little progress in realizing this agenda. In looking at this lack of progress, little attempt has been made to locate the issues on involvement in patient safety in much wider debates about how user involvement has emerged and been addressed in other parts of the public services. More broadly within health and social care, a range of theories and practices have emerged to drive involvement, that draw upon arguments relating to tackling oppressive and discriminatory social structures and health inequalities and power inequities between professionals and service users. These theories provide considerable opportunities for looking at the factors that inhibit involvement and for developing ways that patient and public involvement can best be supported and empowered.

References

Acheson, D. 1998. *Independent Inquiry into Inequalities in Health Report*. London: The Stationery Office.

Adams, R., Dominelli, L. and Payne, M. (eds) 1998. *Social Work – Themes, Issues and Critical Debates*. London: Macmillan.

Allsop, J., Jones, K. and Baggott, R. 2004. Health consumer groups in the UK: a new social movement? *Sociology of Health & Illness*, 26(6): 737–756.

Anderson, P. 2010. Patient safety champions: achievements so far and potential for the future. *Health Care Risk Report*, 16(5): 14–15.

Annandale, E.C. 1989. The malpractice crisis and the doctor–patient relationship. *Sociology of Health and Illness*, 11: 1–23.

Antonsen, S. 2009. Safety culture and the issue of power. *Safety Science*, 47(2): 183–191.

Baggott, R. 2005. A funny thing happened on the way to the forum? Reforming patient and public involvement in the NHS in England. *Public Administration*, 83(3): 533–551.

Barnes, M. 1997. Families and empowerment. In: *Empowerment in Everyday Life: Learning disability*. Edited by P. Ramcharan, G. Roberts, G. Grant and J. Borland. London: Jessica Kingsley, pp. 70–87.

Beresford, P. 2000. Service users' knowledges and social work theory: conflict or collaboration? *British Journal of Social Work*, 30(4): 489–503.

Beresford, P. 2003. User involvement in research: exploring the challenges. *Nursing Times Research*, 8(1): 36–46.

Blane, D. 1991. Health professions. In: *Sociology as Applied to Medicine, 3rd edn*. Edited by G. Scambler. London: Baillièrc Tindall, pp. 221–235.

Braye, S. 2000. Participation and involvement in social care. An overview. In: *User Involvement and Participation in Social Care. Research Informing Practice*. Edited by H. Kemshall and R. Littlechild. London: Jessica Kingsley Publishers, pp. 9–28.

Braye, S. and Preston-Shoot, M. 1995. *Empowering Practice in Social Care*. Buckingham, Open Uuniversity Press.

Bristol Royal Infirmary Inquiry. 2001. *The Report of the Public Inquiry into Children's Heart Surgery at the Bristol Royal Infirmary 1984–1995*. London: HMSO.

Brown, P. and Zavestoki, S. 2004. Social movements in health: an introduction. *Sociology of Health and Illness*, 26(6): 679–694.

Burns, K. 2008. Canadian patient safety champions: collaborating on improving patient safety. *Healthcare Quarterly*, 11(special issue): 95–100.

Bury M.R. 1986. Social construction and the development of medical sociology. *Sociology of Health and Illness*, 8: 137–169.

Care Quality Commission. 2009. *A New System of Registration*. London: Care Quality Commission.

Charles, C., Gafni, A. and Whelan, T. 1999. Decision-making in the physician patient encounter: revisiting the shared treatment decision-making model. *Social Science and Medicine*, 49: 651–661.

Colin-Thomé, D. 2009. *Mid Staffordshire NHS Foundation Trust: A Review of Lessons Learnt for Commissioners and Performance Managers Following the Healthcare Commission Investigation*. London: Department of Health.

Conrad, P. and Leiter, V. 2004. Medicalization, markets and consumers. *Journal of Health and Social Behaviour*, 45: 158–176.

Conrad, P. 2005. The shifting engines of medicalization. *Journal of Health and Social Behaviour*, 46: 3–4.

Cooper, L., Coote, A. and Davies, A. 1995. *Voices Off? Tackling the Democratic Deficit in Health*. London: Institute for Public Policy Research.

Coulter, A. and Ellins, J. 2006. *Patient-Focused Interventions A Review of the Evidence*. London: Picker Institute.

Cowden, S. and Singh, G. 2007. The 'user': friend, foe or fetish?: A critical exploration of user involvement in health and social care. *Critical Social Policy*, 27(5): 5–23.

Dalrymple, J. and Burke, B. (eds) 2006. *Anti-Oppressive Practice – Social Care and the Law*. Maidenhead: Open University Press.

Davies, H.T.O. and Shields, A.V. 1999. Public trust and accountability for clinical performance: lessons from the national press reportage of the Bristol Hearing. *Journal of Evaluation in Clinical Practice*, 5(3): 335–342.

Davis, R.E., Jacklin, R., Sevdalis, N. and Vincent, C.A. 2007. Patient involvement in patient safety: what factors influence patient participation and engagement? *Health Expectations*, 10(3): 259–267.

Department of Health 1990. National Health Service and Community Care Act 1990. London: HMSO.

Department of Health. 1991. *The Patient's Charter*. London, HMSO.

Department of Health. 1999. *Patient and Public Involvement in the New NHS*. London: Department of Health.

Department of Health. 2000. *The NHS Plan*. London: The Stationery Office.

Department of Health. 2003a. *Strengthening Accountability: Involving Patients and the Public*. London: Department of Health.

Department of Health. 2003b. Health and Social Care (Community Health and Standards) Act. London: Stationery Office.

Department of Health. 2006. *A Stronger Local Voice: A Framework For Creating a Stronger Local Voice in the Development of Health and Social Care Services*. London: Department of Health.

Department of Health. 2007. *World Class Commissioning*. London: Department of Health.

Department of Health. 2008a. *High Quality Care For All: NHS Next Stage Review Final Report*. London: Department of Health.

Department of Health. 2008b. *Real Involvement: Working With People To Improve Services*. London: Department of Health.

Department of Health. 2008c. *Stronger Voice, Better Care*. London: Department of Health.

Department of Health. 2009. *Tackling Concerns Locally – Report of the Clinical Governance Subgroup*. London: Department of Health.

Department of Health. 2010a. *The NHS Constitution*. London: Department of Health.

Department of Health. 2010b. *Equity and Excellence: Liberating the NHS*. London: Department of Health.

Department of Health. 2010c. *Liberating the NHS: Report of the Arm's-length Review*. London: Department of Health.

Disability Rights Commission (DRC). 2005. *Equal Treatment: Closing the Gap*. London: Disability Rights Commission.

Donaldson, L. 2008. The challenge of quality and patient safety. *Journal of the Royal Society of Medicine*, 101: 338–341.

Dyer, C. 2007. Bill to abolish patients' forums criticised as 'disgraceful'. *British Medical Journal*, 334(7586): 177.

Fallowfield, L. 2010. Communication with patients after errors. *Journal of Health Services Research and Policy*, 15(1): 56–59.

Fleming-Carroll, B., Matlow, A., Dooley, S., McDonald, V., Meighan, K. and Streitenberger, K. 2006. Patient safety in a pediatric centre: partnering with families. *Healthcare Quarterly*, 9(Special Issue): 96–101.

Friedson, E. 1970. *Professional Dominance: The Social Structure of Medical Care*. Chicago, IL: Aldine Publishing Company.

Gabe, J., Bury, M. and Elston, M.A. 2005. *Key Concepts in Medical Sociology*. London: Sage Publications.

Healthcare Commission. 2009. *Listening, Learning, Working Together?* London: Healthcare Commission.

Hogg, C.N.L. 2007. Patient and public involvement: what next for the NHS? *Health Expectations*, 10(2): 129–138.

House of Commons. 2009. *Patient Safety – Sixth Report of Session 2008–2009*. London: The Stationery Office.

Illich, I. 1974. Medical nemesis. *The Lancet*, 1(7863): 918–921.

Illich, I., Zola, I.K., McKnight, J., Kaplan, J. and Shaiken, H. 1977. *Disabling Professions*. London: Marion Boyars Publishers.

Irvine, D. 2004. *The Doctors' Tale*. London: Routledge.

Kennedy, I. 2003. Patients are experts in their own field. *British Medical Journal*, 326(7402): 1276–1277.

Kings Fund. 2006. *Access to Health Care for Minority Ethnic Groups*. London: Kings Fund.

Kohn, L.T., Corrigan, J.M. and Donaldson, M.S. 1999. *To Err Is Human: Building A Safer Health System*. Washington, DC: National Academies Press.

Leape, L.L., Berwick, D.M. and Bates, D.W. 2002. What practices will most improve safety?: evidence-based medicine meets patient safety. *Journal of American Medical Association*, 288(4): 501–507.

London Health Observatory (LHO). 2005. *Indications of Public Health in the English Regions*. London: London Health Observatory.

Marmott Review, The. 2010. *Fair Society, Healthy Lives*. London: The Marmott Review.

McLean A. 1995. Empowerment and the psychiatric consumer/ex-patient movement in the United States: contradictions, crisis and change. *Social Science and Medicine*, 40(8): 1053–1071.

Mid Staffordshire NHS Foundation Trust Inquiry. 2010. *Independent Inquiry into Care Provided by Mid Staffordshire NHS Foundation Trust*. London: The Stationery Office.

Mulcahy, L. 2000. Threatening behaviour? The challenge posed by medical negligence claims. *Current Legal Issues*, 3: 82–105.

NHS Executive. 1999. *Clinical Governance in the New NHS*. London: NHS Executive Quality Management Branch.

NHS Management Executive. 1992. *Local Voices: The Views of Local People in Purchasing for Health*. Leeds: NHS Management Executive.

National Audit Office. 2003). *Achieving Improvements through Clinical Governance*. London: National Audit Office.

National Audit Office. 2007. *Improving Quality and Safety: Progress in Implementing Clinical Governance in Primary Care. Lessons for the New Primary Care Trusts*. London: National Audit Office.

National Audit Office. 2008. *Feeding Back? Learning from Complaints Handling in Health and Social Care*. London: National Audit Office.

National Association of LINk Members. 2011. *Healthwatch: Making It Happen – A NALN Report*. London: National Association of LINk Members.

National Leadership Council. 2010. *The Health NHS Board – Principles for Good Governance*. London: National Leadership Council.

Nettleton, S. 1995. *The Sociology of Health and Illness*. Cambridge: Polity Press.

Newell, S.M., Jones, D.A. and Hatlie, M.J. 2010. Partnership with patients to improve patient safety. *Medical Journal of Australia*, 192(2): 63–64.

Oakley, A. 1976. Wisewoman and medicine man: changes in the management of childbirth. In: *The Rights and Wrongs of Woman*. Edited by J. Mitchell and A. Oakley. Harmondsworth: Penguin, pp. 17–58.

Ocloo, J. 2008. Towards partnership: patient and public involvement in patient safety. *Health Care Risk Report*, 14(5): 15–17.

Ocloo, J. 2010. Harmed patients gaining voice: challenging dominant perspectives in the construction of medical harm and patient safety reforms. *Social Science and Medicine*, 71: 510–516.

Parliamentary and Health Service Ombudsman. 2011. *Report of The Health Service Ombudsman on Ten Investigations into NHS Care of Older People*. London: Parliamentary and Health Service Ombudsman.

Parsons, S., Winterbottom, A., Cross, P. and Redding, D. 2010. *The Quality of Patient Engagement and Involvement in Primary Care*. London: The King's Fund.

Parsons, T. 1951. *The Social System*. New York: Free Press.

Peat, M., Entwistle, V., Hall, J., Birks, Y. and Golder, G. 2010. Scoping review and approach to appraisal of interventions intended to involve patients in patient safety. *Journal Health Services Research and Policy*, 15(1): 17–25.

Perrow, C. 1984. *Normal Accidents: Living With High Risk Technologies*. Princeton, NJ: Princeton University Press.

Pickard, S., Marshall, M. and Rogers, A. 2002. User involvement in clinical governance. *Health Expectations*, 5(3): 187–198.

Reason, J. 1997. *Managing The Risks of Organizational Accidents*. Aldershot: Ashgate.

Rogers, A. and Pilgrim, D. 1991. Pulling down churches: accounting for the British mental health users' movement. *Sociology of Health and Illness*, 13(2): 129–148.

Royal Liverpool Children's Inquiry. 2001. *The Royal Liverpool Children's Inquiry Report*. London, HMSO.

Rutter, D., Manley, C., Weaver, T., Crawford, M.J. and Fulop, N. 2004. Patients or partners? Case studies of user involvement in the planning and delivery of adult mental health services in London. *Social Science and Medicine*, 58: 1973–1984.

Schon, D.A. 1983. *The Reflective Practitioner: How Professionals Think in Action*. London: Temple Smith.

Sharpe, V.A. and Faden, A.I. 2001. *Medical Harm*. Cambridge: Cambridge University Press.

Shipman Inquiry Website. 2001–2005. http://www.the-shipman-inquiry.org.uk, accessed 22 March 2011.

Silbey, S.S. 2009. Taming prometheus: talk about safety and culture. *Annual Review of Sociology*, 35: 341–369.

Summerton, J. and Berner, B. (eds) 2003. *Constructing Risk and Safety in Technological Practice*. London: Routledge.

Starkey, F. 2003. The professional and liberational perspectives in social care. *Social Policy and Society*, 2(4): 273–284.

Tait, L. and Lester, H. 2005. Encouraging user involvement in mental health services. *Advances in Psychiatric Treatment*, 11: 168–175.

Timmermans, S. and Berg, M. 2003. *The Gold Standard*. Philadelphia, PA: Temple University Press.

Taussig, M.T. 1980. Reification and consciousness of the patient. *Social Science and Medicine*, 14b: 3–13.

Townsend, P., Davidson, N. and Whitehead, M. 1988. *Inequalities in Health: The Black Report and the Health Divide*. London: Penguin.

Tritter, J.Q. and Lester, H. 2007. Health inequalities and user involvement. In *Challenging Health Inequalities*. Edited by E. Dowler and N. Spencer. London: The Policy Press, pp. 175–192.

Vincent, C., Taylor-Adams, S. and Stanhope, N. 1998. Framework for analysing risk and safety in clinical medicine. *British Medical Journal*, 316: 1154–1157.

Vincent, C.A. and Coulter, A. 2002. Patient safety: what about the patient? *Quality and Safety in Health Care*, 11: 76–80.

Vincent, C. 2006. *Patient Safety*. London: Elsevier.

Warren, J. 2007. *Service User and Carer Participation in Social Work*. Exeter: Learning Matters Ltd.

Warwick, P. 2006. *The Rise and Fall of the Patient Forum. Working Paper No. 25*. York: University of York.

WHO (World Health Organization). 2005. *World Alliance For Patient Safety Forward Programme*. Geneva: World Health Organization.

WHO (World Health Organization). 2007. *European Regional Patients For Patient Safety Workshop Report*. Geneva: World Health Organization.

WHO (World Health Organization). 2008. *Neglected Health Systems Research: Governance And Accountability*. Geneva: World Health Organization.

WHO (World Health Organization). 2010. *Patients for Patient Safety Programme: Impact Analysis*. Geneva: World Health Organization.

Wright, T. and Treacher, A. 1982. *The Problem of Medical Knowledge: Examining The Social Construction of Medicine*. Edinburgh: Edinburgh University Press.

PART 2
Clinical Practice

Chapter 3

Narrowing the Gap Between Safety Policy and Practice: The Role of Nurses' Implicit Theories and Heuristics

Anat Drach-Zahavy and Anit Somech

In May 2009, the following story hit the headlines in the Israeli media, sparking public interest in patient safety. The headline screamed: 'Why was the nurse not forced to take precautions and was allowed to continue handling patients?':

> Hospital regulations require health care employees to take annual screening for tuberculosis. A nurse working in an internal medicine unit in a hospital took the test and discovered that she was carrying the bacterium. She decided not to reveal this fact, took no treatment and continued working at the unit for almost a year. When a patient hospitalized at the unit became infected, she unintentionally revealed that she was actively sick. The nurse was immediately relieved from work and began taking medication. Diagnostic exams at the unit revealed that the nurse had infected four more health care workers. When asked why she had not taken any preventive care, the nurse answered that she knew that preventive treatment could have prevented the eruption of the illness but had decided against taking it as 90 per cent of infected tuberculosis patients do not become actively ill.

(Drach-Zahavy and Somech, 2010: 1406)

Cases such as this, which repeatedly attract public interest around the globe, demonstrate the gap between patient safety policy and practice. Statistics drawn from the US Institute of Medicine show the magnitude of the problem: despite remarkable progress in health care technology and delivery, too many patients apparently die or are injured in consequence of medical errors. In the USA alone, at least 44,000 people, and perhaps as many as 98,000 people die in hospitals each year as a result of medical errors that could have been prevented (Institute Of Medicine 1999). During the years 2000–2002, an average of 195,000 people in the USA died due to potentially preventable, in-hospital medical errors (Health Grades 2004).

One in five Americans (22 percent) reveal that they or a family member has been subjected to a medical error of some kind. This translates into an estimated

22.8 million people in the USA with at least one family member who have experienced a mistake in a doctor's office or hospital (Commonwealth Fund 2002). Based on the Institute of Medicine's (IOM) lower estimate of 44,000 deaths annually, medical errors rank as the eighth leading cause of death in the USA – higher than motor vehicle accidents (43,458), breast cancer (42,297), or AIDS (16,516) (Agency for Healthcare Research and Quality 2003).

Another example of safety violations leading to injuries is hospital-acquired infections. According to the Center for Disease Control and Prevention, in American hospitals alone, hospital-acquired infections account for an estimated 1.7 million infections and 99,000 associated deaths each year (Patient Safety Focus 2001). Moreover, 5–10 percent of the patients who are admitted to US acute-care hospitals acquire one or more infections there, and the risks have steadily increased in recent decades (Burke 2003). These worrying statistics raise three fundamental facts:

1. safety guidelines exist;
2. health care staff are familiar with them;
3. sometimes they decide to ignore them.

In this chapter, we address the question of why, despite enormous investments in developing clear policy guidelines and best practices for addressing safety issues, health care staff still decide to cut corners, and fail to comply with safety regulations. We do so by integrating two lines of research: psychological research on heuristics in the individual's decision-making process, and organizational safety literature.

This chapter elucidates the gap between policy and practice in patient safety. First we present our theoretical framework, before extrapolating this to our empirical findings which illustrate nurses' decision-making processes that discourage safety behaviour. Our main argument is that nurses apparently act according to heuristics leading them to cut corners, thus ignoring safety rules and procedures prevalent in their unit. Following this, taking an organizational perspective, we propose managerial approaches aimed at changing nurses' decision processes and at directing more attention to safety issues.

Understanding Nurses' Safety Behaviour: the Role of Heuristics in Making Decisions

Safety in the health care industry means the avoidance, prevention and amelioration of adverse outcomes or injuries stemming from the processes of health care (Katz-Navon et al. 2005). Such outcomes include errors and accidents caused by treatment actions (in contrast to disease complications), equipment failure, disregard of safety rules and procedures, non-completion of an intended action (for example, surgical events, events involving devices, patient protection and care) and executing the wrong plan for a given aim (Gaba 2000, Leape 2002, Katz-Navon et al. 2005). In this chapter we refer specifically to the safety behaviours of health care staff, which are intended to protect patients directly and indirectly.

Although safety is an organizational issue, bedside health care workers provide care for patients, so it makes sense to explore the question of safety at the individual level. In constructing our argument, it is not our purpose to ignore the Institute of Medicine's conclusion that 'to err is human' (Kohn et al. 1999) by blaming the individual closest to the incident (for example, bedside nurse, physician). Instead we identify human heuristics that typically evolve in situations of limited resources (Kanfer and Ackerman 1989). This comes at a time of emerging consensus that successful safety initiatives will depend on a theoretically sound understanding of employees' perceptions, cognitive processes and heuristics (Leliopoulou et al. 1999, McDonald et al. 2006).

The heuristic method is used to rapidly reach a solution that it is hoped will be close to the best possible outcome or the optimal solution. A heuristic is a rule of thumb, an educated guess, an intuitive judgement, or simply common sense. In more precise terms, heuristics stand for strategies using readily accessible, though loosely applicable, information to solve problems (Pearl 1983). Heuristics are simple, efficient rules, hard-coded by evolutionary processes or learned, which have been proposed to explain how people make decisions, arrive at judgements and solve problems, typically when facing complex problems or incomplete information. These rules work well under most circumstances, but in certain cases lead to systematic errors or cognitive biases (Kahneman 2003).

Based on empirical evidence, we suggest that nurses have developed heuristics as to when and how to follow safety policies, guidelines and rules (Drach-Zahavy and Somech 2010). Our findings highlight that although nurses' non-adherence to safety rules might seem random, it is in fact systematic and predictable. Many of their deviations from safety procedures have stemmed from the uncritical use of implicit theories, heuristics, rules of thumb and self-assessments that lead to biased decision-making in day-to-day conduct in the unit (Henriksen and Dayton 2006). These observations were obtained from a qualitative study, which used a multi-method approach including semi-structured interviews (perceptions), observations (real-time behaviour) and documentary evidence. The sample consisted of nurses from 15 nursing units (internal, geriatric and paediatric wards) in four hospitals in the north of Israel. In each unit, four to seven nurses were interviewed and observed. Because of the complexity and breadth of the data collected, we endeavoured to sample diverse hospitals and nursing units to capture the phenomenon across a specific context. Theoretical saturation was achieved after investigating 15 nursing units.

We found that nurses develop five heuristics for when and how to follow safety procedures. Our first heuristic, *the show must go on*, refers to nurses' internalized instruction to continue caring for patients even at the price of harm to themselves or their patients. This particular source of sub-optimality in behaviour is sometimes called melioration (Herrnstein et al. 1993), meaning to choose the alternative in a set of alternatives that has the current highest yield in utility. This process is often characterized by failure to consider the effect of present choices on future yields. Melioration can thus be thought of as involving a within-person externality, or 'internality', which occurs when one discounts or ignores the consequences of one's own behaviour for oneself. The internality can occur for a variety of reasons: lack of awareness of the consequences, ignorance of how to respond to it, or a motivational downgrading of time-deferred or otherwise obscure consequences of action.

Nurses acting by this implicit rule tend to weigh up the pros and cons of deviating from safety procedures when handling patients, and ascribe top priority to the continuous care for patients. Nurses expressed their commitment to patients not only in emergency situations but also during daily work at the unit. They frequently weighed the risks involved in not protecting themselves, against those involved in continuing the care for patients while unprotected. The following example underscores this motif in the nurses' decision-making processes:

> In an emergency, you're not exactly thinking about gloves, you just get on with the job and take care of the patient. This is your instinct. It is unconscious. If you see a patient in distress, you immediately approach him, and do what is necessary to provide care. If you get pricked in the process, then so be it. In these situations, you think more about how to save the patient than how to protect yourself.

> Nurse, internal medicine ward.

The consequences of not wearing personal protection equipment themselves and not ensuring that their patient did so were deferred despite the risk of harm, whereas the consequences of not continuing the patient's care (for example, working at a slower pace, overloading colleagues) were more proximal. Nurses often chose to cut corners, ignore safety procedures and continue caring for patients without taking the necessary precautions. Another consideration expressed by the nurses was the (in)convenience of using personal protective equipment:

> Under some circumstances, I do not wear gloves, even though I know I should. For example, when taking urine and excrement tests, you need to conduct the test, transfer the secretion to the test tube, write the note, and so forth. Gloves are inconvenient, especially when working with small children. So I often leave the gloves off. It is more efficient like this. Gloves are really inconvenient to work with.

> Nurse, pre-natal ward.

Again, the nurses seemed to weigh the convenience of working without personal protective equipment, which facilitated their providing patients with quality care, against the risk it carried to themselves. Here too, care for patients received priority. Similar findings emerged from an observational study of medication administration safety with nurses (Drach-Zahavy and Pud 2010). In this study we observed the medication administration process in a sample of 173 nurses working in 32 surgical and internal nursing units, recruited from three of the largest hospitals in Israel. In each unit, all head nurses, together with all registered nurses who worked on the morning shift at least three times a week and administered medication, participated in the study. Nurses on the morning shift were chosen to control for the effect of different rosters on Medication Administration Errors (MAEs) (Armitage and Knapman 2003). To do so, we developed a nine-column structured observation sheet for the nine important steps in the medication administration process, based on best practices and Israeli Health Ministry guidelines:

1. physician's prescription of medication;
2. prescription documentation in the cardex (nurses' reporting sheet), preparation of the medication for a specific patient;
3. bedside patient identification before administration of the drug;
4. taking relevant measurements (for example, blood pressure);
5. giving information about the medicine;
6. giving the medicine;
7. making sure that the medicine has been fully taken;
8. signing the cardex to confirm administration of the medication;
9. checking for possible side effects.

Our findings indicated that 63 percent of the nurses did not furnish any information to the patient concerning the medication, as prescribed by the medication administration procedure; and almost all nurses (98 percent) did not check about the occurrence of possible side effects. Although these deviations from procedure in themselves do not necessarily produce adverse consequences for the patient, they create conditions conducive to such consequences. When approached, the nurses explained that when they have to consider their priorities under the overload circumstances typical of today's health care system, it was unnecessary and even redundant to replicate these procedures at each administering of medication, when they had previously given the medication to the patient, without any adverse events or outcomes. Consequently, they felt that there was no need to repeat these procedures (Drach-Zahavy and Pud 2010).

These findings indicate that in contrast to the notion that nurses are reluctant to comply with procedures owing to ignorance and lack of awareness of risks or safety procedures (Leliopoulou et al. 1999), they in fact derive a sense of competence and professionalism from their ability to continue caring for patients even at the risk of unfavourable consequences. Safety rules might be overlooked because of individual workers' sense of personal competence in coping with existing systems. Tucker and Edmondson (2002) concluded that nurses' decision-making appeared to be reinforced by a work context that encouraged them not to divert their attention from the primary task of patient care, and to utilize quick solutions for working around system aberrations.

Arguably, not dwelling on unanticipated events, such as being actively sick with tuberculosis or HIV, serves as a coping mechanism for nurses to manage the personal toll imposed by these events. Expressions such as 'you have to move on' and 'you mustn't let things get to you' might reflect a way of containing these events while needing to move forward and help other patients. If so, it is somewhat disturbing that coping mechanisms to psychologically protect the individual also serve to impede organizational efforts to improve occupational safety (Henriksen and Dayton 2006).

Our second heuristic, *professionals do not seek help*, reflects nurses' need to present themselves as self-reliant and fully capable of working independently, without colleagues' assistance. For example, a nurse might prefer to follow their intuition concerning a course of care rather than consulting with the ward sister or matron, even though they acknowledge that person's expertise. Another example is nurses' preference to lift a heavy patient themselves, without a colleague's help, even though they are aware of the potential musculoskeletal injuries that they might experience as a result of such handling. We found that staff perceived complying with safety rules to be bothersome, because it often meant waiting for a colleague's assistance and increased their dependence on others, with consequent risk to their professional reputation. In the next example, a nurse lifted a heavy patient alone, without using elevating aids. When confronted, he admitted preferring to risk his own safety to avoid having to interrupt colleagues' work:

> This is a large, crowded unit. All the nurses are busy with their patients. Calling someone to help me will take time – from both me and my colleague. I examined the patient and saw that I could lift him alone. I am new in the unit, and have to prove that I can work independently of others. I do not want to show my colleagues that I need help.

> Nurse, orthopaedic unit.

This heuristic was also exemplified in Tucker and Edmondson's (2002) study of patient safety, which showed that nurses' decision-making seemed reinforced in a work context that encouraged them to work as independently as possible, even at the price of reaching less satisfactory solutions. Similarly, our findings show that complying with safety rules is considered bothersome because it often requires waiting and increases the nurses' dependence on others, resulting in risking their professional reputation. Consequently, nurses preferred to work independently even at the risk of harming themselves.

Social support literature is abundant on the potential social cost of seeking help. It highlights its negative effect, as it is experienced as potentially stigmatizing and a threat to the worker's self-esteem and public image (Drach-Zahavy 2004). These social costs include disturbing colleagues by taking up their time or giving them extra work, the threat of losing status, the threat of becoming stigmatized, harm to self or public image, and an admission of inadequacy (Drach-Zahavy 2008). Research has indicated that the higher the perceived cost of seeking support, the less assistance the workers seek, with the obvious result of receiving less help (Anderson and Williams 1996). However, such self-reliance and individual problem-solving efforts work against organizational efforts to implement safety rules.

Our third heuristic directing nurses' decisions as to following or not following safety guidelines is '*it can't happen to me*'. Nurses noted that their experience, professional judgement and competence might immunize them against risks, so they could safely continue providing care while deviating from safety rules and procedures:

> My immune system is strong enough. I do not need protection. The protection is aimed at preventing patient-to-patient infection, not at us. A healthy person's immune system is strong enough.

> Nurse, internal medicine ward.

This motif in nurses' decision-making is in line with the self-serving bias, namely individuals believe that good fortune that comes their way is somehow deserved on account of their good qualities and skills, and is therefore justified (Henriksen and Dayton 2006). Additional evidence of a self-serving bias can be found in studies where large majorities of people claimed to have above-average intelligence (Wylie 1979), or ethics and performance at work (Heady and Wearing 1987), while being oblivious to the 50 percent of the population that fall on the other side of the bell curve. In our study, nurses argued that they sometimes decided not to wear protection when taking blood tests because of their strong immune system or blood test hours. They explained that safety procedures exist mainly for novices; more senior nurses could rely on their experience:

> I am very experienced with these kinds of tests. I have many 'sugar test hours'. I know how to work carefully, and I am sure that I am professional enough to avoid any accidents.

> Nurse, surgical ward.

Nurses believed that their (above-average) health, expertize or professional judgement would guard them against the risk factors in their work, so they did not need to adhere to safety rules and procedures. The problem, of course, is that when people minimize their role in adverse events and exaggerate their role in successful events, they are perpetuating a falsehood. This behaviour also matches the 'proficiency trap' (Tucker and Edmondson 2002, Ramanujam and

Goodman 2003, Drach-Zahavy and Somech 2006), of the relatively non-vigilant behaviour of experts (as compared with novices). Experts who have worked in unsafe conditions, with no adverse consequences, may become overconfident and continue to behave in the same unsafe manner. As a result, nurses might have incorrectly learned to accept such deviations from safety procedures as normal and failed to see the need for corrective actions (Tucker and Edmondson 2002, Ramanujam and Goodman 2003).

Our fourth heuristic affecting nurses' decision processes, *the recency effect*, is the prevalence of an inverted U-shaped accumulation of safety behaviours (Tversky and Kahneman 1973). These authors showed that individuals judge the frequency of an event according to how readily available it is for recall. For example, after an accident occurred, attention was riveted on guarding against its recurrence in the unit:

> After a needle-stick case in the unit, everybody abides by the safety rules, and uses personal protection equipment. However, after a few days, nurses return to their former habits, they leave needles in undesignated places, and do not use gloves and other protective measures while taking blood tests, and so forth.
>
> Senior Nurse, internal medicine ward.

Nevertheless, because of the relatively small number of serious adverse events in any individual unit, as well as a general under-reporting of such events, many nurses did not perceive the occupational safety problem as relevant to them. They tended to judge certain events to be frequent or infrequent, based on how easily they could recall specific examples. This led to an increase in safety behaviours immediately following an accident, soon followed by a fade-out effect. If relatively infrequent events that harm patients or nurses go unreported and are not openly discussed, they remain unavailable. Not surprisingly nurses do not evaluate accurately the potential health hazards embedded in their job (Leliopoulou et al. 1999). Still, infrequent vivid events carry a strong emotional impact because of their tragic nature and their recent occurrence, and are more available for recall. In that case the effect is likely to be overestimated, increasing the likelihood of compliance with safety rules. This can explain why numerous safety interventions, such improvement of hand hygiene, using safety protection equipment, adherence to medication administration procedures – all aimed at protecting patients and care providers – succeed only for a limited time, with a fade-out effect shortly after.

Our fifth and last heuristic is *act safely only when others are watching*. As one nurse noted:

Nurses usually tend to adhere more to safety rules when the head nurse is around or when students are present in the unit. It's the responsibility of the head nurse to make sure that staff-nurses use personal protection equipment.

Nurse, internal medicine ward.

This finding is in keeping with social facilitation theory (Zajonc 1965, Baron 1986), which asserts that the presence of others (especially significant others such as direct supervisors or team members) facilitates adherence to social standards and goals, unlike situations in which the individual works alone. In nurses' decision-making this motif of charging the ward sister or matron to enforce safety procedures is in line with previous research that revealed the narrative identity of professionals: professionals by definition are those who do not follow procedures; management must both follow and reinforce procedures (McDonald et al. 2006). Yet the ward sister or matron cannot be constantly present in the unit and observe all nurses, so enforcement is naturally somewhat sporadic, which in turn can raise issues of unfairness and subsequently resentment. All in all, the narrative of protect yourself only when others are watching contributes to noncompliance with safety procedures.

This notion was also exemplified in our study of medication administration errors (Drach-Zahavy and Pud 2010). We found that of the nine mandatory steps in the medication administration process, four are consistently performed by all nurses with negligible deviations from the procedure: physician's prescription of medication, documenting the prescription in the cardex (nurses' reporting sheet), medicine provision and signing on the cardex to confirm execution. This is not surprising given that all these steps (except medication provision) have to be documented, so are easily supervised by the hospital management. As for medication provision, nurses seem to perceive providing the patient with the medication under the proper conditions as the essence of their professional responsibility. Deviation from procedure regarding this step was rare, but it was quite frequent in respect of steps that are less easily monitored (identifying the patient by name prior to medication provision, taking relevant measures, informing the patient about the medication and checking possible after effects).

In sum, nurses seem to possess adequate knowledge of the occupational risk hazards embedded in their job. However, in attempting to cope with the complex work environment, constrained by high demands, low staffing and multi-tasking, nurses, like other decision-makers, have developed implicit theories of whether or not to comply with safety rules, which have gradually substituted the formal rules. These implicit rules seemed to be further reinforced by personal, social and contextual factors in the unit, limiting the likelihood that the decision-makers (nurses) will discover the fallacy of their behaviour (see Figure 3.1). This raises the issue of how organizations can help nurses acknowledge these fallacies, and hence behave more safely.

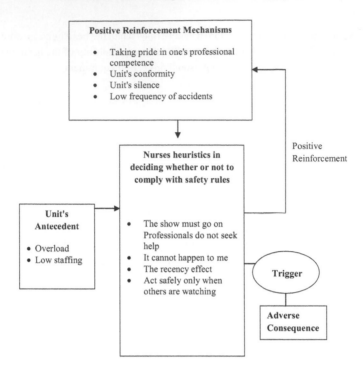

Figure 3.1   Positive reinforcement loops rewarding nurses' heuristics
Adapted from Drach-Zahavy and Somech (2010:1415).

Towards a Safer Workplace: an Organizational Approach to Understanding and Overcoming Nurses' Heuristics

The discussion so far has focused on individual nurses making a decision on whether or not to comply with safety policy and procedures, and on the role of heuristics in this process. However, individuals who either comply or fail to comply with safety policy and procedures do not do so in a vacuum; the organizational context in which these nurses act undoubtedly serves to encourage or discourage them. In the reality of current health care organizations, the common thinking seems to entail that errors = fatal errors (Edmondson 2002). Accordingly, it is not surprising that nurses do not view cutting corners as problematic, and that slight deviations from safety policies are accepted in the overloaded, stressed and multi-task health care environment.

Evidence suggests that 79 percent of adverse consequences for patients (such as severe harm or even death) were attributable to such deviations from standard procedures of medication administration (Fuqua and Stevens 1988, Armitage and Knapman 2003). The false thinking that errors = fatal errors constitutes fruitful ground for our heuristics to grow. To combat it, health care organizations should change the current organizational discourse by reframing the meaning of error from catastrophe to any deviation from standard procedure. This will affect what nurses pay attention to, how they process it and how they strive to maintain constant alertness (Vogus and Welbourne 2003).

However, it is not just front-line clinical staff that are faced with this situation. Managers should also take several steps to cope with the specific heuristics identified. First, the *show must go on* heuristic is reinforced by personal and social factors in the unit, limiting the likelihood that the decision-makers (nurses) will discover the fallacy of their behaviour. Unsafe behaviour is often more attractive, and hence outweighs the expected utility of safe behaviour in the long run. That is, the immediate costs of safe behaviour, such as slower pace, extra effort, or personal discomfort, are given greater weight than low-probability long-term benefits (Zohar and Luria 2004). Moreover, deviating from safety policies and procedures but being an efficient nurse who is able to provide care for patients on time, and saving lives in emergency situations, reinforces the nurse's professional efficacy and competence. Taking pride in one's competence serves as an immediate reward for compromising on safety issues. The negative reward stemming from the possibility of harm to patients is more remote, and is thus less reinforcing.

Moreover, the social environment apparently reinforces the heuristic of *the show must go on*. Nurses, like other individuals working in teams, look to others as valuable sources of information and behavioural guidance (Aronson 1999). If they perceive that physicians or other staff members do not comply with the safety rules, and prefer to press ahead with the care process, they will tend to conform to this norm. Conformity is abetted under several circumstances: when staff members wish to gain acceptance in a group, especially if the group is composed of experts and when a knowledge differential exists between the target person and certain members of the group; or when the group is important to the target person, who will identify more readily with group members (Henriksen and Dayton 2006). Thus, nurses' tendency to comply with the implicit *the show must go on* rule is reinforced by professional and social norms embedded at the health care organizations' culture.

Breaking these positive reinforcement loops can be achieved by assimilating the safety climate as a source of consensual behaviour–outcome expectancies (Zohar 1980, 2000) that serve as cognitive determinants of motivation level (Vroom 1964, Bandura 1986). Safety climate means shared perceptions of work environment characteristics as they pertain to safety matters that affect a group of individuals (Zohar and Luria 2005). Safety climate is expressed and operationalized by supervisory practices. When a consistent pattern of action in regard to safety is displayed, especially when safety considerations conflict with speed or efficiency, it promotes shared perceptions in the group as to the priority of safety (Zohar 2000). Safety climate informs nursing staff of the probable consequences of working safely, and clarifies safety-related management expectations (Zohar 2002). Because human behaviour is primarily responsible for occupational accidents (National Safety Council 1999), a positive safety climate offers a motivational counterweight to the tendency to unsafe action in routine work (Zohar and Luria 2004).

Regarding the second heuristic, *professionals must work alone*, again this seems reinforced by professional values prevalent in many nursing units. Health care organizations are considered an industry context in which individual heroism and skills are assumed to be the critical determinants of important outcomes (Edmondson 2002, Drach-Zahavy 2004). In consequence, self-reliance and autonomy become salient values directing nurses' behaviour, which sends a clear message to staff that seeking help is unprofessional (Drach-Zahavy 2004). Nurses often evaluate their potential gains from seeking help (better safety for patients) against potential losses (being considered unprofessional), and the perceived high social costs outweigh the expected gains from seeking help. As a result, nurses keep working independently, even at the cost of potential harm to themselves and their patient.

To tackle this heuristic, managers should gradually generate a narrative of professionals as those who ask questions, and seek and provide help, rather than those who have all the answers and work independently. Supportive actions by managers can play a key role by modelling support behaviour, thereby contributing indirectly to the creation of a more supportive environment. Nursing managers can also set the ground rules for engaging in support, demonstrate supportive roles and highlight employees' expectations (Drach-Zahavy 2004). This may contribute to the creation of a supportive environment in which nurses feel free to seek the necessary support for delivering quality care.

Another way to promote help-seeking and collaboration in the unit is by creating a work environment characterized by psychological safety. This is a shared belief that well-intentioned interpersonal risk-taking will not be punished (Edmondson 1999). A sense of psychological safety makes it easier to face potentially disturbing or embarrassing outcomes of inquiry, exposure of transparency and the risks of accountability (Hofman and Stetzer 1998, Lipshitz et al. 2002). Managers can foster a sense of psychological safety in nursing staff by encouraging interaction and information exchange in an tolerant atmosphere, sending a clear message that 'you can say anything and will not be judged'. Moreover, nursing staff should experience a clear sense of influence, namely their suggestions and feedback are taken seriously, and are considered in the managers' decision-making. Edmondson (1999) found that psychological safety increases nurses' willingness to report their mistakes, which in turn enhances patient safety and team performance.

Regarding the *it can't happen to me* and the *recency effect* heuristics, because non-adherence to safety procedures does not generally lead to serious accidents, many nurses do not acknowledge the fallacy of these heuristics, and mistakenly perceive their implicit theories as correct. Moreover, organizational silence, or the collective-level feature of doing or saying very little in response to serious organizational problems (Morrison and Milliken 2000), such as occupational safety, allows even the infrequent accidents to be swept under the carpet. According to the management literature, employees decide whether to raise issues with management by 'reading the context' for clues on context favourability (Morrison and Milliken 2000). A favourable context is when nurses perceive the management to be willing to listen and be supportive, and that error reporting has relatively few negative consequences. In general however, underreporting of adverse events indicates that nurses perceive their organizations' context as unfavourable. An unfavourable context is characterized by the shared beliefs that speaking up about problems in the organization is not worth the effort, and that voicing one's opinions and concerns imperils one's job (Naveh et al. 2006). Incidents not acknowledged or brought out into the open cannot be addressed. Consequently, the fallacy exposed as the *recency effect*, and the *it can't happen to me* heuristic, cannot be detected.

To contain these heuristics, it is fundamental that health care organizations be more preoccupied with failure, treating any failure or near miss as a measure of the system's reliability and health, and reward error reporting (Weick 1999). Preoccupation with failure means operating in persistent awareness of the possibility of unexpected events that may jeopardize safety, and engaging in proactive and pre-emptive analysis and discussion. By enhancing the transparency of these infrequent events, organizational silence on them can be countered. Individuals' susceptibility to vividness and recent effects facilitates their being used to advantage to turn the spotlight onto events that might otherwise go unnoticed. Discussions of near misses and accidents, regardless of their actual likelihood, at staff meetings and through written protocols and informal storytelling, will increase the salience of the events and the perceived risks (Henriksen and Dayton 2006). Another means to improve the subjective lens through which nurses evaluate themselves is prompt, objective feedback that is difficult to deny (Henriksen and Dayton 2006). This means that objective feedback on errors should be available to nurses, preferably on the spot, and discussed in team meetings, so that errors will be more visible, and the frequency of such errors will not be underestimated.

Finally, as for *act safely only when others are watching* heuristic, again the organizational context acts as a reinforcement. In health care organizations, efforts to maintain patient safety typically focus on the role of repetition and routine. In such bureaucratic settings nurses frequently perceive that safety is the responsibility of the managers, while their primary focus is on the continuing the care for patient (Henriksen and Dayton 2006). They adhere to safety rules and procedures only when others, particularly the matron or sister, are watching. This pattern of safety behaviours may also exact a price from the unit: lower probability of true learning and implementation of change, factors which were consistently found in earlier research as a potent means to increase patient safety (Edmondson 2002). We found that units that rarely implemented team learning and relied mainly on the supervision of matrons and sisters exhibited higher rates of medication administration errors due to shifting attention to actions that were supervised, while cutting corners with those that were not (Drach-Zahavy and Pud 2010). This heuristic is also reinforced by the perceptions of power differences in the unit. Previous research demonstrated how such power differences become potent inhibitors of learning in teams (Nembhard and Edmondson 2006). For example, 13 percent of medication errors were identified as such through team learning (Drach-Zahavy and Pud 2010). This exemplifies the current perception of learning in health care as a relatively structured activity undertaken by individual practitioners as they prepare to enter independent practice, and later, as they maintain and update their clinical skills (Tucker and Edmondson 2002).

To overcome this heuristic, managers should shift the responsibility for safety from the team leader to team members, by assimilating practices of team learning. This will require a change from a top-down policy of safety encouragement to a bottom-up approach, which empowers bedside nurses to manage safety. Team learning is a process of improving team actions through better knowledge and understanding (Argyris and Schön 1978, Edmondson 2002). Moreover, it is assumed here that a team 'learns' through actions and interactions among people who are typically situated in smaller groups or teams (Edmondson 2002). To promote team learning in the unit, it is necessary to develop structures for learning as well as to assimilate team learning values (Lipshitz et al. 2002). Structures for learning consist of institutionalized structural and procedural arrangements, and informal systematic practices that allow teams systematically to collect, analyse, store, disseminate and use information relevant to the performance of the organization and its members (Lipshitz et al. 2002). Examples are preparatory practice sessions (Edmondson 2002), forms of after-action (or post-project) review (Di Bella et al. 1996), periodic reviews, reviews of statistical indicators of effectiveness (Popper and Lipshitz 2000) and barcode medication administration (Patterson et al. 2004).

Learning values are likely to produce commitment to corrective action:

- *Valid information*: the requirement of complete, undistorted and verifiable information;
- *Transparency*: willingness to hold oneself (and one's actions) open to inspection in order to receive valid feedback;
- *Issue orientation*: evaluation of information strictly on its merits without regard to irrelevant attributes such as social standing of its source or recipient;
- *Accountability*: holding oneself responsible for one's actions and their consequences and for learning from these consequences.

Research has shown that high- and low-learning teams differ by the extent that these four norms are widespread in them (Unger and Erez 2002). All in all, a team-learning approach to promote safety suggests that learning mechanisms set the stage for members to focus attention on deviations from standard procedures and errors, to reflect on them and initiate steps to correct them, preventing them in the future. Learning values ensures that members can openly and trustfully report, discuss and reflect on these errors. When such an approach is integrated into the unit's routine life, nurses will perceive safety as part of their in-role behaviour, and therefore adhere to safety rules regularly, rather than only when supervised.

Conclusion

This chapter integrates two lines of research to better understand the gap between safety policy and practice: psychological research on heuristics in the individual's decision-making process, and organizational safety literature. We identified five specific heuristics which influence nurses' decision not to comply with safety policies and procedures. The organizational literature served as a framework for explaining how these heuristics are strengthened. We described how these heuristics are embedded in the professional and organizational contexts of health care organizations, creating positive reinforcement loops that inhibit nurses' ability to discover the fallacy of their behaviour. Integrating these two lines of research allowed us to offer managerial approaches to combat these heuristics. Specifically, we suggest that safety could be promoted by:

- Assimilating a safety climate.
- Changing the narrative prevalent among nurses for who is a professional nurse, from one who works independently, knows all the answers, and does not need to consult with others, to one who seeks and provides help.
- Promoting psychological safety.
- Treating any failure or near miss as an indicator of the reliability and health of the system.
- Institutionalizing learning practices and values that promote team learning.

By bridging the heuristic and organizational levels, this chapter generates a plethora of new questions and challenges for safety researchers, and also promotes a host of new management issues. Specifically, researchers should embrace a multilevel perspective for addressing the issue of safety in health care organizations. Adopting such a research framework could examine the extent to which the organizational context (for example, norms, organizational structure and values) reinforces the nurse reliance on heuristics in their decision-making on whether to comply or not comply with safety rules. For example, such research can examine whether managerial practices such as safety climate, team learning and psychological safety matters for limiting the occurrence of heuristics. We believe that adopting this framework can provide further insights into how to narrow the gap between safety policy and practice in current health care organizations.

References

Agency for Healthcare Research and Quality, 2003. *AHRQ Annual Report on Research and Financial Management, FY 2002.* AHRQ Publication No. 03-0013. Rockville, MD: U.S. Department of Health and Human Services, Agency for Healthcare Research and Quality.

Anderson, S. E. and Williams, L. J. 1996. Interpersonal, job, and individual factors related to helping processes at work. *Journal of Applied Psychology*, 81(3), 282–296.

Argyris, C. and Schon, D. 1978. *Organizational Learning: A Theory of Action Perspective*. Reading, MA: Addison-Wesley.

Armitage, G. and Knapman, H. 2003. Adverse events in drug administration: a literature review. *Journal of Nursing Man*agement, 11, 130–140.

Aronson, E. 1999. *The Social Animal*, 8th edn. New York: Worth Publishers.

Bandura, A. 1986. *Social Foundations of Thought and Action*. Englewood Cliffs, NJ: Prentice Hall.

Baron, R. A. 1986. Distraction-conflict theory: progress and problems. In: *Advances in Experimental Social Psychology*, edited by L. Berkowitz. Orlando, FL: Academic Press, pp. 1–40.

Burke, J. P. 2003. Infection control – a problem for patient safety. *The New England Journal of Medicine*, 348, 651–656.

Commonwealth Fund. 2002. *Improving the Quality of Healthcare Services. 2002 Annual Report*, pp. 33–43. New York: Commonwealth Fund.

DiBella, A. J., Nevis, E. C. and Gould, J. M. 1996. Understanding organizational learning capability. *Journal of Management Studies*, 33(3), 361–379.

Drach-Zahavy, A. 2004. The proficiency trap: how to balance enriched job designs and the team's need for support. *Journal of Organizational Behaviour*, 25, 979–996.

Drach-Zahavy, A. 2008. Workplace health friendliness: a test of a cross-level model. *Journal of Occupational Health Psychology*, 13(3), 197–213.

Drach-Zahavy, A. and Somech, A. 2006. Professionalism and helping: harmonious or discordant concepts? An attribution theory perspective. *Journal of Applied Social Psychology*, 36(8), 1892–1923.

Drach-Zahavy, A. and Somech, A. 2010. Implicit as compared with explicit safety procedures: the experiences of Israeli nurses. *Qualitative Health Research*, 20, 1406–1417.

Drach-Zahavy, A. and Pud, D. 2010 Learning mechanisms to limit medication administration errors. *Journal of Advanced Nursing*, 66(4), 794–805.

Edmondson, A. C. 1999. Psychological safety and learning behaviours in work teams. *Administrative Science Quarterly*, 44, 350–383.

Edmondson, A. C. 2002. The local and variegated nature of learning in organizations: a group-level perspective. *Organization Science*, 13, 128–147.

Fuqua, R. and Stevens, K. 1988. What we know about medication error: a literature review. *Journal of Nursing Quality Assurance*, 3(1), 1–17.

Gaba, D. M. 2000. Structural and organizational issues on patient safety: a comparison of health care to other high-hazard industries. *California Management Review*, 43(1), 83–102.

Heady, B. and Wearing, A. 1987. The sense of relative superiority central to well-being. *Social Indicators Research*, 20, 497–516.

HealthGrades. 2004. *HealthGrades Quality Study: Patient Safety in American Hospitals*. Lakewood, CO: HealthGrades, Inc.

Henriksen, K. and Dayton, E. 2006. Public policy and research agenda: organizational silence and hidden threats to patient safety. *Health Services Research*, 41, 1539–1554.

Herrnstein, R. J., Loewnstein, G. F., Prelec, D. and Vaughan, W. 1993. Utility maximization and melioration: internalities in individual choice. *Journal of Behaviour and Decision Making*, 6, 149–185.

Hofmann D. A. and Stetzer, A. 1998. The role of safety climate and communication in accident interoretation: implications for learning from negative events. *Academy of Management Journal*, 41(6), 644–656.

Institute of Medicine 1999. *To Err is Human: Building a Safer Health System*. Washington, DC: National Academy Press.

Kahneman, D. 2003. Maps of bounded rationality: psychology for behavioral economics. *The American Economic Review*, 93(5), 1449–1475.

Kanfer, R. and Ackerman, P. L. 1989. Motivation and cognitive abilities: An integrative/aptitude-treatment interaction approach to skill acquisition [monograph]. *Journal of Applied Psychology*, 74, 657–690.

Katz-Navon, T., Naveh, E. and Stern, Z. 2005. Safety climate in health care organizations: a multidimensional approach. *Academy of Management Journal*, 48, 1075–1089.

Kohn, L. T., Corrigan, J. M. and Donaldson, M. S. (Eds). 1999. *To Err is Human: Building a Safer Health System*. Washington, DC: Institute of Medicine, National Academy Press.

Leape, L. L. 2002. Reporting of adverse events. *New England Journal of Medicine*, 347, 1633–1638.

Leliopoulou, C., Waterman, H. and Chakrabarty, S. 1999. Nurses failure to appreciate the risks of infection due to needle stick accidents: a hospital based survey. *Journal of Hospital Infection*, 42, 53–59.

Lipshitz, R., Popper, M. and Friedman, V. J. 2002. A multifacet model of organizational learning. *The Journal of Applied Behavioural Science*, 38, 78–98.

McDonald, R., Waring, J. and Harrison, S. 2006. Rules, safety and the narrativisation of identity: a hospital operating theatre case study. *Sociology of Health and Illness*, 28(2), 178–202.

Morrison, E. and Milliken, F. 2000. Organizational silence: a barrier to change and development in a pluralistic world. *Academy of Management Review*, 25(4), 706–725.

National Safety Council. 1999. *Injury Facts*. Itasca, IL: National Safety Council.

Naveh, E., Katz-Navon, T. and Stern, Z. 2006. Readiness to report medical treatment errors: the effects of safety procedures, safety information, and priority of safety. *Medical Care*, 44, 117–123.

Nembhard, I. M. and Edmondson, A. C. 2006. Making it safe: the effects of leader inclusiveness and professional status on psychological safety and improvement efforts in health care teams. *Journal of Organizational Behaviour*, 27(7), 941–966.

Patient Safety Focus. 2001. *Patient Safety: Current Statistics*. Online: Patient Safety Focus: A patient safety resource focused on information, programs and solutions. Available at: http://www.patientsafetyfocus.com/patient-safety-current-st.html, accessed 16 February 2011.

Patterson, E. S., Rogers, M. L. and Render, M. L. 2004. Fifteen best practice recommendations: recommendations for bar-code medication administration in the Veterans Health Administration. *Journal of Community Quality and Safety*, 30(7), 355–365.

Pearl, J. 1983. *Heuristics: Intelligent Search Strategies for Computer Problem Solving*. New York: Addison-Wesley.

Popper, M. and Lipshitz, R. 2000. Organizational learning mechanisms, culture, and feasibility. *Management Learning*, 31, 181–196.

Ramanujam, R. and Goodman, P. S. 2003. Latent errors and adverse organizational consequences: a conceptualization. *Journal of Organizational Behaviour*, 24, 815–836.

Rogers, B. 1997. As I see it. Is health care a risky business? *The American Nurse*, 29, 5–6.

Tucker, A. L. and Edmondson, A. C. 2002. Managing routine exceptions: a model of nurse problem solving behaviour. In: *Advances in Healthcare Management*, edited by G. T. Savage, M. D. Fottler and J. D. Bair. New York: JAI Press/Elsevier, pp. 87–113.

Tversky, A. and Kahneman, D. 1973. Availability: a heuristic for judging frequency and probability. *Cognitive Psychology*, 5, 207–532.

Unger-Aviram, E. and Erez, M. 2002. Goal orientation and learning values: their effects on regulatory processes and learning at the individual and team levels. Invited Symposium on Work Motivation. XXV International Congress of Applied Psychology (ICAP), Singapore, July, 2002.

Vogus T. J. and Welbourne T. M. 2003. Structuring for high reliability: HR practices and mindful processes in reliability-seeking organizations. *Journal of Organizational Behaviour*, 24, 877–903.

Vroom, V. H. 1964. *Work and Motivation*. New York: Wiley.

Weick, K. E. 1999. Improvisation as a mindset for organizational analysisis. *Organization Science*, 9(5), 543–555.

Wylie, R. 1979. *The Self-Concept: Vol. 2. Theory and Research on Selected Topics*. Lincoln, NE: University of Nebraska Press.

Zajonc, R. B. 1965. Social facilitation. *Science*, 149, 269–274.

Zohar, D. 1980. Safety climate in industrial organizations: theroetical and applied implications. *Journal of Applied Psychology*, 65(1), 96–102.

Zohar, D. 2000. A group-level model of safety climate: testing the effect of group climate on micro-accidents in manufacturing jobs. *Journal of Applied Psychology*, 85, 587–596.

Zohar, D. 2002. The effects of leadership dimensions, safety climate, and assigned priorities on minor injuries in work groups. *Journal of Organizational Behaviour*, 23, 75–92.

Zohar, D. and Luria, G. 2004 Climate as a social-cognitive construction of supervisory safety practices: scripts as proxy of behaviour patterns. *Journal of Applied Psychology*, 82, 322–333.

Zohar, D. and Luria, G. 2005. A multilevel model of safety climate: cross-level relationships between organization and group-level climates. *Journal of Applied Psychology*, 90, 616–628.

Chapter 4

Resources of Strength:
An Exnovation of Hidden Competences to
Preserve Patient Safety

Jessica Mesman

Today's health care system involves many practices that are highly complex and involve a host of activities that are embedded in tightly knit infrastructures. Many of the daily activities are marked by a high level of interdependency and require a high level of specialization of clinicians. Because of the prominent role of interactive complex technologies, the intensity of the work and the potential of catastrophic consequences, these practices are referred to as 'high-3 work environments': high-tech, high-intensity and high-reliability (Owen et al. 2009).[1] Critical care practices like the Emergency Department (ED), the Operating Room (OR) and the Intensive Care Unit (ICU) are vivid examples of high-3 work environments. What they have in common is the potential of major incidents with drastic consequences on an everyday basis. As a consequence of the real-time nature of the work, events must be managed while evolving. Once a procedure is initiated, it cannot be stopped. This creates a strong sense of urgency and time-pressure. Since errors may lead to unacceptable and irreversible consequences, high-3 work environments involve risky practices that call for a maximal degree of safety. However, several studies – most prominent amongst them the one of the Institute of Medicine in the United States of America (Kohn et al. 1999) – have shown an unacceptably high level of adverse events and near-misses.[2] This has prompted the rise of a global patient safety movement.

---

1 Besides health care many practices can be characterized as high-3 work environments. They can be found in, for instance, the aviation and chemical industry and nuclear power plants.

2 Error rates also proved to be high outside the United States. For instance, in their review about the scale and nature of adverse events in British hospitals, the Department of Health (2000) reports that at least 850,000 patients are involved in incidents per year. This figure reflects 10 per cent of all annual hospital admissions in the UK. The additional costs are estimated to amount to £2 billion. The latest study on incident rates in the Netherlands shows that 2.3 per cent (30,000 people) of the overall patient population was involved in unintended incidents, one third of which will suffer lasting consequences. Besides the devastating consequences for patients and their families and the loss of trust in the health

Using the expertise of other high-risk industries, the main strategy in health care is learning from mistakes. As such, most safety initiatives are geared towards prevention of adverse events by detecting and eliminating causes of error. Much attention is given to developing blame-free reporting systems of incidents and mistakes, electronic patient records with a built-in warning system, training to enhance teamwork and ways to diffuse best practices and cultivate safety cultures. However, as outlined in the introduction of this volume, mainstream patient safety research is uncritical of the current prevailing ideas in health care policy. Its scope, as argued by Rowley and Waring (see the Introduction to this volume), is too narrow and its presumptions about health care practices are too simple as it completely ignores the local specificity of the complexity of health care situations.

Indeed, the analytical scope of today's patient safety research is too narrow, as most studies on patient safety are geared towards the causes of errors and as such towards the absence of safety. Complementary to this approach, I would like to propose a research perspective that focuses on the presence of safety and explores its texture. After all, the realization of a sound and safe practice is not only based on error-reducing activities, but also on a sophisticated understanding of the vigour of health care practices. In this chapter I will therefore outline an alternative research agenda which concentrates on the resources of safety, notably the informal or unarticulated ones. My exploration of latent resources can be considered as a form of exnovation. Exnovation refers to the attempt to foreground what is already present – though hidden or overlooked – in specific practices, to render explicit what is implicit in them (Wilde 2000). In the context of patient safety this attempt is directed at the existing but unnoticed competences and strength of practices that allows them to preserve adequate levels of safety.

A Turn Towards Capabilities

Patient safety research aims to identify and eliminate causes of incidents. The outcomes of these studies form the basis for adjustments in health care practice. These adjustments are implemented through top-down directives in the form of evidence-based standards and protocols. Standardization of practices is at the core of the reorganization of work. In this approach, patient safety is considered a matter of error measurement and management (Rowley and Waring, Introduction to this volume) and all efforts are directed to protect the patient from unreliable actions and decisions on various levels: that of the hospital organization, the ward and the individual doctor or nurse. In doing so, these studies focus on errors and the level of reliability.

Notwithstanding the good intentions of this kind of patient safety research, there is growing criticism of its underlying assumptions about practice, its research

---

care system, the additional financial costs are estimated to be 167 million Euros (de Bruijne et al. 2007).

focus and the implementation of results in a 'one-size-fits-all' form (Grol et al. 2008, Rowley and Waring Introduction to this volume, Iedema et al. forthcoming). Instead of discussing this critique extensively, I would like to direct the attention to one particular aspect in this discussion: the error-focused analysis of most patient safety research.

Béguin et al. (2009) describe how the focus of research into accidents shifted from the individual blame to a more system approach with Reason's (1990) notion of 'latent errors' as one of the core concepts. Subsequently, there was a shift in attention from the investigation of accidents to ways of preventing these errors. Irrespective of the shift from individual to systems, and from accidents to threat reduction, research is, according to Béguin et al., still based on a deficit model.[3] However, there is a growing consensus that error-focused research is inadequate for studying the dynamics and complexities of today's health care practices (Dekker 2006, Vincent 2006, Béguin et al. 2009). Complex sociotechnical work environments, like hospitals, are fallible by their very nature and breakdowns, failures and incidents are an inherent characteristic of their work practices (Summerton and Berner 2003, Owen et al. 2009). This implies that more rules and regulations, protocols and other procedures will never fully eradicate the imperfection of work practices. No matter how many errors are repaired they will inevitably recur in other forms at other times and places. In other words, error-reducing initiatives turn out to be a matter of rearranging vulnerability. Most measures and strategies, rather than diminishing, merely relocate the vulnerability of practices. In this way, vulnerable and risky situations are not removed, but merely moved around (Mesman forthcoming b).

Despite all the efforts to improve patient safety, it is clear for everyone involved that such a goal is hardly a straightforward matter. The level of complexity in health care practices is such that unintended, collateral effects of safety measurements can neither be predicted nor be prevented. There has been a growing awareness that we need to move beyond these 'counting and control' models of thinking if we want to understand safety in such complex sociotechnical work environments like hospitals. Therefore, it is argued, practices should not only be reliable. The reliability position is built on a world of stability. This is, according to Foster (1993), an illusion. The size, complexity, patterns and control structures of today's social-technological practices make them inherently vulnerable and unpredictable. For this reason, it is important to move beyond a focus on individual error and reliability, and acknowledge the multifaceted nature of safety problems. Instead, health care practices should be resilient, that is having the ability to resist disturbances and recover from disruptions because safety is not simply the outcome of a system, but an emergent property (Dekker and Hollnagel.

---

3   Béguin et al. (2009) explain this persistence of error-focused analysis on the basis of the purposes this kind of research can fulfil in terms of accountability (attributing responsibility), learning (from mistakes) and trust (re-establish faith in technology through repair of errors).

2005, Healy and Mesman forthcoming). Safety is not a static feature of a system, but something it may or may not produce. Safety, in other words, is 'a dynamic, interactive, communicative act that is created as people conduct work … and gather experiences from it' (Dekker and Hollnagel 2006: 6).

A conceptualization of 'safety' as an emergent property and of 'practice' as being inherently imperfect is also prompting us to rethink the position of clinicians. If practices are imperfect by nature, we have ample reason to wonder why things do not go wrong more often in these complex care settings. Why are there not more errors and incidents? Critical care settings like ICU's and emergency and surgical departments are especially prone to errors. Considering the high-risk work environments and the vulnerability of their patient population we have reason to expect many more incidents. Following Owen et al. (2009), we can ask ourselves: how are health care practitioners able to produce safe and reliable performances *despite* fallible technologies, sometimes unrealistic rules and incompatible procedures and systems that are inherently imperfect by their very nature? What is done and used to maintain an adequate level of patient safety? This question takes the positive role of clinicians and the environment they work in as point of departure for studying patient safety. Such research has its focus on everyday dynamics instead of the more common (human) error analysis.

Although the significance of a reduction of errors and mistakes is beyond discussion, I would like to argue that defining patient safety as the absence of errors follows from too narrow a focus. Patient safety should be more than the absence of errors and incidents. We should also characterize patient safety on the basis of what it is, instead of what it is not (Dekker 2005). In this perspective the realization and preservation of a sound and safe practice is not only based on the elimination of risks and the absence of errors, but also on strengthening of what is safe already. Accordingly I argue that the identification and understanding of the vigour of health care practices is as important for patient safety as the identification of the patient's and practices' vulnerability. This change of focus will bring other elements of patient safety to our attention and yield another set of questions. These questions will be directed by the ambition to identify the resources used to establish and preserve a sound and safe health care practice. Indeed, we can learn from mistakes, but also from what is done in the right way. Therefore, we should widen our analytical focus and include the fabric of safety itself as well as it is embedded in the basic but sound structure of the health care practice.

Apart from the intended formal measures such as built-in alarm systems and double-checking of medication, patient safety is also achieved by an unplanned and perhaps unarticulated but effective set of actions and initiatives. Maintaining the necessary level of safety requires a circumstantial intervention in which both formal and informal safety activities play a role. Following on from this, studying patient safety should aim to explicate these non-intentionally built-in structures and contextual contingencies that contribute to the constitution of the field. Patient safety research, then, should *not only* focus on the causes of incidents and near-misses, but *also* analyse causes of safety. In doing so one should *not only* focus on explicit, intentional or formal safety measures, such as protocols, guidelines, technological equipment designs and professional knowledge and procedures, but *also* include its informal and implicit resources of strength. The question of which informal resources of strength enable staff members of a health care practice to manage the risks and the unexpected and rise above decision-making dilemmas in order to maintain optimal patient safety, does not imply that formal and evidence-based standards and procedures are ignored. On the contrary, they will not be considered as *the* solution for safety problems, but rather as one of the many ingredients of the fabric of the practice in which patient safety is accomplished.

The research perspective presented in this chapter is in line with the theoretical frame developed in science and technology studies (STS). For one thing, this angle allows for the criticism of the assumption that the fundamental structure of (medical) practice is constituted by principles, deductive patterns of reasoning and decision protocols. Empirical studies of specific practices found no evidence for these assumptions.[4] Instead, detailed studies of medicine-in-action show how day-to-day operations can never be reduced to a mere application of rules and theoretical principles. Knowledge is not simply waiting out there to be applied in practice; it is constituted in the very same practice as it is used. Likewise, safety is not present or absent, but an emergent property. In this perspective, clinical work does not have the sole function of being the context in which busy doctors and nurses are moving around and make their decisions on treatment and prognoses. On the contrary, a turn to practice capitalizes on a careful analysis of the concrete work performed as part of a treatment trajectory. This perspective can provide insight into how knowledge, standards and regulations considering safety are reshaped in the vortex of concrete activities, skills and behaviours involved in the preservation of patient safety.[5]

In sum, the acknowledgement of the imperfection of practices directs us – paradoxically – to move outside the domain of errors. First, it makes us wonder about the causes of safety, instead of incidents and mistakes. Secondly, it redirects our focus away from vulnerability to the vigour of practices. Thirdly, it underlines the significance of the positive contribution of the clinicians in preserving adequate levels of safety. Finally, it also takes into account the informal and implicit resources of safety. In other words, the focus is not on what is absent, but on what is present even if latent – not as latent failures, but as 'latent resources' of safety.

Exnovation: Another Approach to Study Patient Safety

Obviously, a safe and sound performance cannot be explained on the basis of protocols and professional knowledge alone. 'Something more' is involved

---

4   For examples of medicine-in-action: Berg (1997), Berg and Mol (1998), Franklin and Roberts (2006), Goodwin (2009), Lock et al. (2000), Mesman (2008).

5   For a fine-grained analysis of how practitioners rely on different ways of reasoning, acting and interacting, see Mesman (2008).

in engaging in practice than just following the instructions (Lynch 1983: 207). Following Lynch (1983), much of what evidently makes up the orderliness and ordinariness of patient safety is not worth talking about in the idiom of the standardized and the general. Instead 'we should discover and demonstrate the ways in which various [safety] practices compose themselves through the vernacular conversations and the ordinariness of embodied disciplinary activities' (Lynch 1983: 208). It is this 'something more' – this hidden competence – that deserves our attention as well.

What I will pursue can be best described as 'exnovation', a concept coined by Wilde (2000). Exnovation pays attention to the mundane, to the implicit local routines, to what is already in place. In rendering explicit what is implicit, exnovation shares a focus with ethnomethodology. However, exnovation has the explicit aim to improve practices. In this objective it resembles practices of innovation. Where innovation can be simply defined as 'to make something new to improve practices', exnovation pays attention to what is already in place and challenges the dominant trend to discard existing practices in improvement processes (Wilde 2000:13). More than innovation, exnovation does justice to the creativity and experience of the clinicians, in their effort to assert themselves in the particular dynamic of the practice they are involved in. Importantly, 'things or practices are not less valuable simply because they already exist' (Wilde 2000: 13).

In health care this perspective is about foregrounding the manifold resources and skills that clinicians bring to bear on what goes on. It allows the development of a fresh perspective on the competence and ingenuity of the clinicians and the specific structure of their practice (Mesman 2008). In the context of patient safety research exnovation is the explication of hidden competences that constitute the basic fabric of a safe and reliable practice (Iedema et al. forthcoming). Therefore, exnovation uses the creativity and ingenuity of clinicians as point of departure for practice improvement and gives prominence to existing sources of safety.

The analytical scope of exnovation questions dominant ways of understanding safety as defined as the absence of errors and incidents, and offers another perspective on clinicians in regard to patient safety. Starting from the recognition of the competence of clinicians as they assert themselves in the dynamic of complex situations, exnovation considers their accomplishments in everyday practice an extraordinary achievement.

An explication of the ingredients of safety work is relevant for the following reasons. First, it will contribute to the understanding of the actual practice of preserving levels of patient safety. To understand these practices of competence is important, because mere analysis of errors and breakdowns and problem-solving cannot illuminate the full range of elements that contribute to the safety of complex and risky practices. Exnovating these (latent) resources of strength and safety offers insights into clinicians' ability to order the complexity of the day-to-day practice and produce a reliable performance. These coordinative acts of the flux and change of daily practice come with specific modes of ordering (Law 1994). Exnovation elucidates these competencies of co-ordination and the alignment of these modes of ordering of which those involved are not always aware. If theoretical development and practical insights rely on error analysis only, these kinds of accomplishments will always remain a concealed attribute to day-to-day action. Secondly, insight into the kind of adaptive strategies and negotiations that contribute to a reliable performance can be used to enhance professional practices in different ways. By illuminating the strength of practices, opportunities to strengthen what is already strong are opened up. Thirdly, it enriches the conceptualization of patient safety because it provides an image of patient safety that falls outside the scope of incidents and errors. Fourth, an explication of the existing resources of safety will increase clinicians' safety sensibility and capability. Finally, by identifying the locus of strength we can prevent safety measures which are solely based on error analysis destroying perfectly well functioning practices. Implementing these kind of safety measures can seriously interfere with existing but unknown safety practices. Instead of making things safer, perfectly well functioning – but hidden – parts of patient safety work might be weakened or even ruined. An explication of these latent resources of strength can prevent such outcome.

With this approach I deliberately move away from error-focused analysis. Other approaches, like 'resilience engineering' and 'appreciative inquiry' have made the same move based on similar motivations. Resilience engineering is 'a paradigm for safety management that focuses on how to help people cope with complexity under pressure to achieve success' (Woods and Hollnagel 2006: 6). It moves away from error reduction to learning from failure, focuses on problem-solving behaviour and aims to improve the practice in such a way that it becomes 'better able to recognize, adapt to, and absorb disruptions that would otherwise fall outside the base it was designed to handle' (Dekker and Hollnagel 2006: 6). By monitoring and assessing the adaptive capability of an organization, resilience engineering attempts to develop explicit guidance for complex practices on how to make trade-offs between safety and situational pressures, like lack of time or being short of appropriate equipment. Appreciative inquiry equally has its focus on the positive side of inquiry. Appreciative inquiry is 'the art and practice of asking questions that strengthen a system's capacity to apprehend, anticipate, and heighten positive potential' (Cooperrider and Whitney 2005: 11). Its intention is to discover, understand and foster innovations in social-organizational arrangements and processes (Cooperrider and Srivastva 2005). As an affirmative approach, appreciative inquiry also moves away from problem-based management.

Exnovation shares the positive approach of both these approaches. However, unlike resilience engineering, exnovation has no intention to monitor, model, assess and predict effects of change on resilience of organizations. Neither does exnovation share the appreciative inquiry's aim to innovate. This is not to say that exnovation does not aim to improve practices. On the contrary, we should not ignore the lessons we can learn from what is already in place and goes right. For this reason, patient safety research should not only be focused on error analysis and its standardized solutions or resilience but should also include analyses with a focus on existing practical know-how (exnovation) (Iedema et al. forthcoming). In foregrounding collective creative processes, exnovation, in other words, constitutes the necessary complement to resilience and proceduralized solutions.

Exnovation of the texture of safety raises several questions. For instance, do we really know what and why things are going well and secure patient safety? Are we able to recognize the unplanned but effective sets of action? Which structures and processes constitute the fabric of a safe and sound practice? What are the resources involved in the numerous interventions that are performed on a more or less routine basis? Sound answers to these kinds of questions require detailed analysis of the structures and processes as they unfold in the day-to-day routines of practices. However, the question remains *how* to study these issues from the perspective of exnovation. The remainder of this chapter will be devoted to this question. I will begin by discussing two different – though complementary – methodological tracks, first the 'classic' thorough analysis to gain insight and second the collaborative intervention to make a difference. In the next section I will provide some examples of studies of sound and safe practices. But first I will elaborate on these two tracks.

Analysis of Safety

How to study safety outside the domain of errors and incidents? A point of departure is that in this type of research it is not about trouble, mistakes, imperfection, flaws and inadequacies, but about if things are going well, how they are supposed to be, about safe and sound practice. Yet, instead of being 'just' the error-free counterpart, sound practices should be defined on the basis of their own modalities. From this perspective we can regard practices as specific arrangements of processes that constitute the safe and sound texture of the practical order. These arrangements include heterogeneous sets of elements, such as technical and social devices, time and space, people and things, norms and values, formal and informal knowledge, expertise and experience and customs and habits. All these elements constitute the basic fabric of 'normal' practice and therefore should be taken into consideration. Then how to identify the constituents of safety in the regular routines of everyday performance? How to identify the already present but as of yet unrecognized aspects of patient safety? It is easier said than done. To study what is already in place yet hidden is hardly an easy task. To study the hidden competence of practices to maintain patient safety, therefore, first some more reflection on method is called for.

The methodological consequence of a focus on latent resources of safety is threefold. First, to gain insight into these matters we cannot rely on quantitative data collection and analysis. More than quantitative research, qualitative methods such as ethnography are pre-eminently suited for studying the dynamics of safety practices *in situ*. A detailed study of 'sustainable safety' in complex care practices that is based on participant observation provides insight into the way ordinary work processes contribute to patient safety. Secondly, since this kind of research is geared towards the explication of self-evident actions and their potential for safe practice, processes rather than products will be the centre of attention. Moreover, the focus will be on gradualization (alignment, fine-tuning) rather than on a comparative/contrastive approach (for example expertize versus experience). Thirdly, a study of those parts of practice that are not related to errors (elimination) and problems (solving) implies an analytical scope on the ordinary, the usual, the regular, and therefore almost invisible, hard to notice aspects of patient safety. To gain access to the various implicit methods and strategies of preserving patient safety in the day-to-day routines requires special attention to the analytical points of entry.

What then are possible analytical points of entry to study causes of safety in its formal and informal form? Actually, there are different *kinds* of analytical entries. It is possible, for instance, to concentrate on modes of ordering, like clinicians' styles of reasoning and study the different kind of repertoires they use to make their daily decisions (for example Mesman 2008). Secondly, instead of modes of ordering, the practice can be opened up along the line of specific topics, such as handovers, infection prevention or other patient safety-related issues and why they go well. Thirdly, we can also focus on particular practices, such as communicative practices and *in situ* interactions. A fourth option is formative structures of our daily reality such as time and space, which illustrates the spatial and temporal analysis of particular situations in health care practice.

Collaborative Interventions

In following Markussen and Olesen (2007), I reject the repair metaphor. Instead I will try to contribute to the 'safety sensibility' and question dominant ways of understanding safety by using the method of video reflexivity. Video has the ability to capture the details of processes and interactions and is therefore widely used in health research (Lomax and Casey 1998, Xiao and Mackenzie 2004, Forsyth et al. 2009). Besides its more common use of generating data for the purpose of academic analysis, video can also be used for practice change. By using video footage of local practices, clinicians can observe and reflect on their *own* practices, learn from it and if necessary, redesign their practice (Carroll et al. 2008). It is in close collaboration with the clinicians on the ward that the researcher designs the research agenda and identifies specific areas of 'everyday' practices to video-record, which are subsequently explored more closely with clinicians in so-called video-reflexivity meetings.[6] The video footage is edited into short clips, which are then replayed back to the clinicians as feedback sessions. In these sessions clinicians make sense of the data alongside the researcher (Carroll 2009, Iedema

---

6 For a critical reflection on video-ethnography, see Carroll and Mesman (forthcoming).

and Carroll 2010). Video reflexivity as a method provides the possibility that clinicians themselves set out their own trajectories of learning and changing instead of an outsider, like a researcher or a top-down implemented standard procedure that directs the way. These fast feedback methods can lead to new ways of talking, thinking, seeing and doing everyday practice for clinicians and researchers alike (Forsyth 2009, Iedema et al. 2009). In the tradition of the interventionist video-ethnography the method of data collection and reflection on the basis of videos should be considered as 'a product' for clinicians on the ward to be used by them. It provides them a tool to decide for themselves where and how to reorganize their work.

In sum, exnovation patient safety requires a sophisticated understanding of latent resources of safety and 'forums of engagements' where clinicians themselves can think and talk about what they do well (Iedema et al. forthcoming). The remaining part of this chapter will outline some examples of how to study resources of safety. In this exploration of competences I will first focus on the role of spatial order, followed by an analysis of patient safety in relation to the temporal order.

A Methodological Exploration of Exnovation

In the following I will explore different ways to study resources of safety. The neonatal intensive care unit (NICU) can serve as a context for presenting examples of studies on causes of safety. This ward is specialized in the care and treatment of newborns. Very young babies end up in a NICU because their lives are seriously at risk on account of their prematurity, complications at birth, congenital diseases or potentially lethal infections. Needless to say, this vulnerable patient population calls for a high level of patient safety and special care. The interventions necessitate a dynamic, intricate and ongoing fine-tuning of actions and reactions among the individual clinicians, as well as between clinicians and the technology they use. Since this chapter aims to discuss the relevancy of a particular analytical focus – one that includes the unproblematic, the ordinary, the usual, the regular – the empirical data reported have to be considered as illustrations, rather than serving as hard evidence of a fine-grained analysis of hidden competences as such.

I will use the spatial and temporal order of the NICU, respectively, as entry points to articulate the constituents of safety in this practice. Let us start with the spatiality of patient safety research, and how can we think 'geographically' about patient safety (Mesman 2009, Mesman forthcoming a).

A Geography of Patient Safety

An analysis of the spatiality of patient safety requires both a focus on the (coordinating) role of the (material) environment as well as an analysis of the way spatial order is produced by safety activities (Mesman 2009). In other words, in what way does location matter in regard to patient safety? A focus on the spheres of action directs analytical focus to what is actually done in which exact location and how this is related to patient safety. To gain insight into the spatiality of patient safety, I will focus on one specific kind of space: the sterile space, and one specific medical procedure: the insertion of a central venous catheter. Questions to answer are: what, in this procedure, is the role of spatial ordering in maintaining an adequate level of sterility? What is the spatial distribution of activities and attention of the clinicians involved? Do their safety activities bear the imprint of their location? And vice versa, in what ways does sterile work affect the spatial order? Let's take a closer look.

The vulnerability of the newborns on the NICU calls for a strictly controlled environment. However, safety measures are not limited to the architectural design of the ward, such as its airlock at the entrance and the isolation room. A safe space to act in is also accomplished, as I will show, by practices of spatial ordering. To study the role of spatial order in the production of patient safety, a sterile insertion of a central venous catheter will serve as a case study.[7] A central venous catheter is a small tube that is inserted into the baby's bloodstream and provides access to the baby's body to administer medication and nutrition. Although essential for the treatment of these ill babies, a central line is not without risk as it can cause infections. To keep the germs out, clinicians aim to work with sterile instruments in a sterile environment. Based on (video) ethnographic data from research in the Netherlands, I will describe how particular spatial arrangements produce sterility and how, at the same time, sterility work produces specific spatial orders. Sterility is, I argue, all about space. Sterility can be regarded as 'carving out' a specific kind of space: one that is free from infectious micro-organisms.

A NICU is not a sterile space. Therefore it is important to restrict the mobility on the ward of the clinicians and instruments involved. The degree of mobility and the level of sterility are tightly coupled. Anticipating the mobility restriction, a nurse collects all that is needed and positions it next to the incubator of the baby:

> NICU: One of the neonatologists just asked the nurse who is responsible for this morning's new admission, to prepare the insertion procedure they need to do on 'her' patient. Therefore she moves the cart with instruments from the corner of the ward to the incubator. Next an instrument trolley and the folding screens follow. She positions the carts and screens strategically around the incubator. When everything is in place she pulls out a checklist, opens the drawers of the cart and gathers the materials according to the list. The neonatologist – now fully scrubbed, gowned and gloved – joins her in the little space between the incubator and the folding screens and starts to select the items he needs for the insertion of the central line. He carefully arranges all the materials he selected from the sterile set, as well as the items the nurse has placed on the sterile field

---

7 This description is based on ethnographic research in the Netherlands on a NICU where I did participant observation for eight months during spring 2007 and 2008.

on the trolley next to him. However, instead of arranging the instruments in a
haphazard way on the sterile field, the neonatologist orders them carefully.

The excerpt above depicts a reconfiguration of human bodies, pieces of
furniture and sterile equipment. However, on what basis is the situation reordered?
A closer look reveals that, for example, the grouping of items is based on the
interrelationships between the items and on their position in the sequential order
of the medical procedure. What needs to be used first, such as the disinfectant,
is placed within easy reach. They are, in other words, 'assembled in readiness'
(Lynch et al. 1983: 227). With this collecting and ordering of big and small
materials, people and technology an orderly structure is provided that facilitates
the sequential steps to be taken in order to prepare the insertion of the catheter.
The specific compositional order of materials (including the folding screens) and
equipment directs the focus of the attention and the locus of the hands and, as
such, acts as 'an infrastructure of attention' (Mesman 2009: 1709).

After the assembly of pieces of furniture and human bodies around the
incubator, the process of convergence of the spatially distributed resources
continues and shifts into the incubator. With this move, the available space to act
is further reduced from the size of the ward, the space around the incubator and
the sterile field into the interior space of the incubator. Now the activity field is
so small that it only allows room for the hands of the staff and the baby's body.
Performing a medical procedure in this small sterile field involves an aseptic
disciplining that requires a high level of spatial coordination and the capability to
move around in limited space.

The production of sterility involves the relocation of the field of activity,
the assemblage of an infrastructure of attention, the composition of selected
equipment on a sterile field and the scaling down of one's degree of mobility
and range of action. Sterility turns out to be a product of spatial orderings and,
therefore, requires an adequate level of spatial awareness and spatial coordination.
This, however, is just one side of the story, because the production of sterility itself
produces a specific spatial order. Sterility work maps out the ward in a specific way
by producing buffers and boundaries. Sterility and spatial order are co-produced
in the same process.

For example, in preparing to insert a central venous catheter, the spatial order of
the ward is reframed into special zones: clean and dirty places, open and restricted
spaces, spaces where you can move freely and those where you have to stay put,
accessible and inaccessible spaces, and 'private' and 'public' spaces. During the
insertion procedure the boundaries of these disparate domains shift, dissolve and
sometimes reappear. As one of the nurses explains:

> While he (the neonatologist) scrubs in we cannot use that sink. I have to take
> care of Joyce today and the water I need for bathing her or to refill the water in
> her incubator I have to walk to the other side of the room to use the sink over

there. You can imagine that I don't like to do that, but we are all aware that sterility comes first.

Boundaries between, for instance, specific 'open access areas' and 'restricted areas' move from one side of the ward (the sink where the doctor scrubs in) to the other side of the ward (next to the incubator). But the 'private' domain of the neonatologist at the sink dissolves the moment s/he walks away. There is no fixed spatial order. Instead sterility travels from place to place, just like germs. But unlike germs, this journey requires a well-orchestrated 'chain of replacements' from one field of activity to another (Latour 1995: 175).

Yet the spatial order of sterility intersects with the spatial order of other lines of activity: caring practices, therapeutic practices, family practices, dying practices and research practices. When these lines of activity meet, a normative structure becomes visible in what is prioritized. Insight into the normative structure of these co-existing spatial orders turns out to be crucial for patient safety. By analysing processes of spatial fine-tuning in everyday practice, it becomes possible to identify spatial competences and circumstances that enable staff members to provide safe health care. As such, a spatial analysis offers an alternative perspective of patient safety, one that takes into account its spatial dimension. It demonstrates how, besides the content of the formal protocol on the insertion procedure, other modes of knowledge, like spatial competence, and other kinds of concern, like competing lines of activities or navigating through a non-sterile area, play a crucial role in patient safety. In other words, a spatial analysis of sterility demonstrates how space matters in the production and preservation of patient safety. Spatial ordering turns out to be a constitutive part of the accomplishment of sterility. From this perspective, sterility is about carving out a specific space; about creating boundaries and buffers; about staging a trajectory over which sterility can travel from the different corners of the ward all the way into the incubator and into the infant's vein.

In sum, a spatial analysis of patient safety provides another conceptualization of both patient safety and space. Space in this perspective is not the passive environment in which people move around and activities occur, but an active 'doing' that takes part in the constitution of patient safety. By analysing processes of spatial fine-tuning in everyday practice, it becomes possible to identify spatial competences and circumstances that enable staff members to provide safe care. These insights can increase the 'safety sensibility' of clinicians in another way as it offers an alternative image of patient safety, one that takes into account, among other things, its spatial dimension.

Horizons of Expectation

To present another example of a study on causes of safety I will analyse a commonly applied NICU procedure: a tracheal intubation.[8] In case of respiratory trouble, a baby will receive oxygen through an endotracheal tube connected to the respirator machine. Tracheal intubation is the positioning of a tube into the windpipe (trachea), a complex procedure that requires close collaboration. In this case study, the analytical entry point will not be space, but time. What is the role of time in the mechanisms, interventions and processes that are needed to turn a dynamic web of clinicians and others, including the devices and machines, into one single and safe collaborative collective? My analysis suggests that collaborative action relies on a whole body of diagnostic practices. Time is, as I will show, a crucial element in these diagnostic processes. In this analysis the notion of 'time' is used to refer to the interrelationship between past, present and future instead of clock time.

In medical settings 'diagnosis' generally refers to the identification of a disease. Yet diagnosis is also geared to the hazards of medical intervention, and the identification of these problems is at the heart of error prevention. By broadening the analytical scope we can include dynamic diagnosis of how things are going as they are (also when they are going well). This form of diagnosis is about recognition of the overall task structure, the ability 'to read' the conduct of co-participants and the identification of opportunities for actions. Although practices are often critically and pervasively augmented with this 'positive mode' of diagnostic work, it is often invisible and has therefore been under-theorized in medical and nursing literature. By illuminating this kind of work in relation to teamwork, opportunities for strengthening the safety of critical care practices are opened up (Mesman 2010).

The positioning of an endotracheal tube is essential for providing respiratory support. For most NICU patients, respiratory support plays a central role in the treatment. To allow the respirator to insert a mixture of air and oxygen into the lungs of the baby, a tube is inserted into the infant's nose (or mouth), passing the glottis (the space between vocal cords in the voice box) into the windpipe. This procedure cannot be performed by a single person and is quite risky. In a teaching hospital the procedure involves a resident, a supervising neonatologist and two nurses. Considering the risks involved and the collaborative nature of this intervention, this procedure serves as a useful case to demonstrate how diagnostic work is an integral part of safe, collaborative medical practice and how temporal orders are accommodated in this process. A preparatory stage of an intubation procedure involves anticipation of the near future. This is expressed in the assessment of the condition of the baby and the arrangement of the instruments. Before the actual intubation is started, a nurse collects and checks the equipment.

---

8   This case study is based on my study of diagnostic work. For an extended and detailed account see Mesman (2010).

Next the neonatologist and the resident who has to do the actual intubation, double-check the presence and functioning of the equipment. They need to be sure that everything is connected correctly. However, checking equipment is more than just turning switches on and off. A thorough check presumes full understanding of the purpose of instruments, so as to be able to assess their proper working.

> NICU: The neonatologist picks up the laryngoscope and switches its light on and off and hands it over to the resident who is doing the same thing. 'Before you start, always double-check if everything is here and make sure it works. You cannot afford any delay because something is missing or doesn't work.' Next the resident takes the oxygen-bag and squeezes it. Then she picks up the mask and holds it near the baby's face. Together they discuss how to measure the right size of the mask and tube. Then they turn around to check the respiratory machine and the monitor behind the incubator. After being sure everything functions properly the neonatologist switches off the alarm of the monitor: 'let's have some tranquillity over here'.

To be able to enter fully into the complicated task, the environment is accommodated. To avoid a non-stop alarm from sounding and ensure a tranquil environment for the nervous resident, the neonatologist switches off the alarm of the monitor. In this way he tries to create a safe 'infrastructure of attention' (Mesman 2009). As the neonatologist explains:

> The resident has to focus on her task. So, I always speak quietly and turn off the sound of the alarm so the resident is not disturbed by the sound, nor will she look at the monitor. Because that is what they always do: when the alarm goes off, they look up. The resident should also not suction the baby's throat because that is the job of the nurse. She should keep her eyes focused on the tube. In this way I try to create a situation of peace and quietness so the resident can fix her attention to this job.

While doing this the neonatologist and the resident not only double-check the presence and functioning of equipment. Additionally, they also go over the intubation procedure to anticipate the sequence of actions and moments of risks and accommodate the environment to the task ahead. Being aware of the complexity of the procedure, the neonatologist prepares the resident by rehearsing imaginatively the sequential steps and hurdles of the intubation procedure. By envisioning the intubation procedure, the doctors project a scenario of what needs to be done, what the risks are and what to look for. This 'imaginative rehearsal' can be considered as a preparation of the diagnostic work that lies in the immediate future: the work that needs to be done *while* inserting the tube. The envisioned near future does not only involve the risky parts of the trajectory, but also its practical stages and related tasks. By pointing out the specific tasks involved and what cues to look for, the neonatologist aims to direct the diagnostic focus of the resident. Providing a dry run will help the resident to keep paying attention to what happens in and outside the baby's mouth, while focusing on the actual intubation. To support the direction of the focus potential distractions, like the alarm of the monitor above the incubator, are taken away. In this way imaginative rehearsal has to be considered as one of the core elements of safety activities.[9]

Both the imaginary rehearsal of the procedure and the detection of potential distractions involve a form of anticipating that includes more than 'just' what needs to be done. It also involves the diagnostic work that needs to be done during the intubation. In other words, these preparatory activities are aimed at optimizing the diagnostic work that lies ahead in the immediate future. This in itself is a diagnostic activity. It requires, for example, the ability to distinguish between supportive and distractive aspects of the environment.

However, the diagnostic work involved in an intubation procedure is not only directed towards the condition of the newborn or the workings of the instruments. In order to work safely, the various tasks to be undertaken rely on extremely close collaboration. Much of the diagnostic work is aimed at becoming one collaborative intubating ensemble. Collaboration involves the interweaving of sequential and concurrent tasks. All these activities are aimed at performing an intubation as smoothly and safely as possible. Turning this dynamic intertwining into a smooth medical procedure calls for a thorough orchestration that is filled with diagnostic work. A safe and swift intubation will depend on a perfectly timed, close-knit and accurate collaborative effort – on becoming one. In their effort to become one the temporal aspect is crucial since it requires acting in the 'same present'. No one should lag behind or be ahead of the others. Imaginative rehearsal contributes to such a concurrent synchronized performance.

Sociological studies of teamwork stress that collective work formations call for coordinative work. It requires 'the continuous dynamic structuring of people's interactions with each other and with their material environment' (Suchman 1996: 410). Rather than emerging out of the blue, collectives are the product of a specific kind of labour: articulation work (Strauss 1985, Suchman 2000). People apply various mechanisms of interactions to reduce the complexity of a situation and, as such, the overhead costs of articulation work (Schmidt and Bannon 1992). Examples are the organizational structures in the form of formal or informal allocation of responsibilities and the use of treatment plans and protocols.

In medical practice, protocols function as a classic example of these articulation resources. A protocol functions as a 'focal point of reference to which different staff members refer, can orient themselves, and can find instructions on what to do next' (Berg 1998: 232). As Suchman (1987) pointed out, plans and protocols are just resources for situated action. They do not tell us what to do in a specific situation, since no formal description can be so complete that it can

---

9 Imaginative rehearsal is not only related to safety issues. Clinicians do rehearse possible futures while confronting ethical dilemmas as well. See Coeckelbergh and Mesman (2008).

deal with local circumstances which bring in unexpected contingencies. To get the job done, no matter the circumstances, implies a compromise that resolves these problems. Nevertheless, protocols play an important part in collaborative efforts as 'mechanisms of interaction in the sense that they reduce the complexity of articulating cooperative work' (Schmidt and Bannon 1992: 19). In performing their tasks doctors and nurses delegate part of their coordinating activities to protocols. In other words, a protocol acts as a collaborative resource for the orientation of routine connections between tasks and activities. It provides a basis for reading certain forms of conduct or courses of actions as it projects subsequent actions (Hindmarsh and Pilnick 2002).

However, protocols also play an important role in anticipating the future. Although both doctors and nurses have their own responsibilities and protocols, in the case of intubation the nursing protocol is designed within the medical frame of reasoning. The overlap with the medical protocol is striking indeed, as it refers to medical indications, contraindications and medical complications. Strictly speaking, it cannot be considered as a nursing protocol. After all, nurses have to deal with objectives, indications and complications tied to their own specific role and expertise. According to one of the nurses:

> Normally the objectives of our protocols are aimed at supporting the doctors or related to specific care activities. However, in this particular case the objective of our protocol is the same as that of the doctor's; that is the optimalization of the respiratory function of the baby. Overlap is crucial in this case since no one involved can afford staying one step behind. We anticipate the same kind of things. We have to because there is simply no time to do one more step if immediate action is called for. I am where the doctor is. We walk the way together, so to say. I can think along with him since my actions are almost based on the same protocol.

The protocols act as an anticipative resource (Mesman 2010) that assist clinicians in linking up ongoing actions with what comes next in a smooth way. A protocol helps them to read the embodied conduct of their colleagues as well as to see the same future, and subsequently it acts as a resource for organizing their work seamlessly (Hindmarsh and Pilnick 2002). In its current form the nursing protocol enables the nurse to look through the eyes of her medical colleague and vice versa, when assessing the situation. Coherency of anticipation is crucial for coherency of actions. The unity of nursing and medical protocols results in a shared perspective and matching anticipation, thus facilitating tight coupling of actions. Any difference between the two protocols would require demand time to understand how the two can be combined. However, this is time which is unlikely to be available when a patient is unwell.

What does this example tell us about exnovation and patient safety? The analysis of the role of anticipation in an intubation procedure on a NICU contributes to our understanding of diagnostic work in collaborative practices.

A large proportion of diagnostic work includes also seeing the opportunities for action within sequences of collaborative practice, and these opportunities are not necessarily remedial actions. Insights in anticipative resources contribute to our understanding of successful collaboration. Mostly, collaboration is considered as solely a matter of working together. A closer look at daily activities, though, reveals a rich repertoire of anticipative work. To be a collective requires not only the ability to recognize the overall structure of work in the here and now, but also in the immediate future. One needs to know what to expect and recognize potential for problems *and* opportunities for action and resources for support.

Since anticipative skills are crucial for the articulation work that collaboration demands, training programmes for clinicians should acknowledge this aspect of diagnostic skill. Additionally, an increasing awareness of the scope of diagnostic activities and the diagnostic ability to recognize resources including those that lie ahead in the immediate future will contribute to the level of patient safety. Patient safety is not only about noticing trouble and adequate and accurate practices in the present, but also in what comes next. Be ready for it. Not just to avoid failures, but also to grasp opportunities when they are there. Be ready for them as well.

Concluding Remarks

Nowadays, there is a growing recognition in risk and safety studies that errors and problems should be considered as part of the natural state of practices. The starting point in these studies is the reliable performance of practitioners despite the imperfect work environment. These kinds of studies move away from the error paradigm and turn their focus on the positive side of practices. Aiming to enhance the adaptive capabilities of organizations they focus on the learning capabilities of practitioners. However, their desire to shift the focus beyond errors could not prevent that 'such analyses have often still remained centred on the loss of comprehension or the failure' (Béguin et al. 2009: 4). Therefore I propose another approach to patient safety, one that moves away from errors and their solutions, and turns towards what is going well and is already in place. In this respect, the argument of this chapter explores the possibility of a better understanding of patient safety by analysing the strength of practices and their (latent) resources for safety.

It is argued that patient safety research needs to widen its analytical scope and include research projects that study the selecting and combining of different platforms of action. This raises questions about the locus of strength in practices. What informal measures and initiatives contribute to a high level of patient safety? What is the role of the staff members' own situated rationalities in relation to the framing of safety? Which informal modes of knowledge are involved in the preservation of patient safety? By analysing processes of fine-tuning different modes of knowledge in day-to-day routines of work, it becomes possible to identify competences that enable staff members to provide safe and sound health care.

Results of these kinds of studies can open up new opportunities for reinforcing what is already strong. As such this study has to be considered as critical towards yet complementary to deficit-based studies.

To gain insight into the available resources of strength it proved to be methodologically productive to focus on the spatial and temporal order of practice. On the basis of participant observation in a NICU I have provided a sketch of two studies that investigate the safe and sound fabric of its everyday practice. For example, using the spatial order as analytical entry point I identified processes of continuous relocation of activity fields, the assemblage of an infrastructure of attention, the composition of selected equipment, and the scaling down of one's degree of mobility and range of action as they are enacted in daily work processes. Likewise, an analysis of the temporal order of their procedures foregrounds the significance of anticipation and imagination as being crucial for a preservation of patient safety.

Whereas clinicians are trained to identify problems, it is much more difficult to unravel one's own latent resources of strength. Most of the time, for instance, clinicians hardly realize that they are using processes of imaginative rehearsal as a tactic. Also, collaboration is considered as just a matter of working together. A closer look at their daily activities, though, reveals a rich repertoire of informal reasoning, genres of acting and communicating. Patient safety research that is aimed at an explication of those implicit processes can contribute to the clinicians' ability to identify resources of strength and recognize the different modes of action. Degrees of mobility, genres of simplification, modes of anticipation and other supportive resources deserve as much attention as troubles, errors and incidents. Or, put differently: reliable and adequate processes are as worthy of scholarly scrutiny as disturbing ones and this needs to be recognized as an important focus of study.

References

Béguin, P., Owen, C. and Wackers, G. 2009. Introduction: shifting the focus to human work within complex socio-technical systems. In: C. Owen, P. Béguin and G. Wackers, eds, *Risky Work Environments. Reappraising Human Work Within Fallible Systems*. Aldershot: Ashgate, pp. 1–10.

Berg, M. 1997. *Rationalizing Medical Work: Decision Support Techniques and Medical Practices*. Cambridge, MA: MIT Press.

Berg, M. 1998. Order(s) and Disorder(s): of protocols and medical practices. In: M. Berg and A Mol, eds, *Differences in Medicine: Unraveling Practices, Techniques, and Bodies*. Durham, NC: Duke University Press, pp. 226–243.

Berg, M. and Mol, A. (Eds) 1998. *Differences in Medicine: Unraveling Practices, Techniques and Bodies*. Durham, NC: Duke University Press.

Carroll, K. 2009. Insider, outsider, alongsider: examining reflexivity in hospital-based video research. *International Journal of Multiple Research Approaches Approaches*, 3, 246–263.

Carroll, K. and Mesman, J. (forthcoming). Ethnographic context meets ethnographic biography: a challenge for the mores of doing fieldwork. *Journal of Multiple Research Approaches*.

Carroll. K., Iedema, R. and Kerridge, R. 2008. Reshaping ICU ward round practices using video-reflexive ethnography. *Qualitative Health Research*, 18, 380–390.

Coeckelbergh, M and Mesman, J. 2007. With hope and imagination: imaginative moral decision-making in neonatal intensive care units. *Ethical Theory and Moral Practice*, 10, 3–21.

Cooperrider, D. L. and Srivastva, S. 2005. Appreciative inquiry in organizational life. In: D. L. Cooperrider, P. F. Sorensen, T. F. Yaeger and D. Whitney, eds, *Appreciative Inquiry: Foundations in Positive Organization Development*. San Francisco, CA: Berret-Koehler Publishers, pp. 61–104.

Cooperrider, D. L. and Whitney, D. 2005. A positive revolution in change: appreciative inquiry. In D. L. Cooperrider, P. F. Sorensen, T. F. Yaeger and D. Whitney, eds, *Appreciative Inquiry: Foundations in Positive Organization Development*. San Francisco, CA: Berret-Koehler Publishers, pp. 9–34.

Dekker, S. 2005. *Ten Questions about Human Error: A New View of Human Factors and System Safety*. London: Lawrence Erlbaum Associates.

Dekker, S. 2006. *The Field Guide to Understanding Human Error*. Aldershot: Ashgate.

Dekker, E. and Hollnagel, E. 2005. *Resilience Engineering: New Directions for Measuring and Maintaining Safety in Complex Organizations*. Lund: Lund Universitet, Linköping Universitet, The Ohio State University.

Dekker, S. and E. Hollnagel. 2006. *Resilience Engineering: New Directions for Measuring and Maintaining Safety in Complex Systems*. Lund: Lund University.

Department of Health. 2000. *An Organization with a Memory*. London: TSO.

Forsyth, R. 2009. Distance versus dialogue: modes of engagement of two professional groups participating in a hospital-based video ethnographic study. *International Journal of Multiple Research Approaches*, 3, 276–289.

Forsyth, R., Carroll, K. and Reitano, P. 2009. Introduction: illuminating everyday realities: the significance of video methods for social science and health research. *International Journal of Multiple Research Approaches*, 3, 214–217.

Foster, H. D. 1993. Resilience theory and system evaluation. In: J. A. Wise, V. D. Hopkin and P. Satger, eds, *Verification and Validation of Complex Systems: Human Factors Issues*. Berlin: Springer-Verlag, pp. 35–60.

Franklin, S. and Roberts, C. 2006. *Born and Made: An Ethnography Of Pre-Implantation Genetic Diagnosis*. Princeton, NJ: Princeton University Press.

Goodwin, D. 2009. *Acting in Anaesthesia: Ethnographic Encounters With Patients, Practitioners And Medical Technologies*. Cambridge: Cambridge University Press.

Grol, R., Berwick, D. and Wensing, M. 2008. On the trail of quality and safety in health care. *British Medical Journal*, 336, 74–76.

Healy, S. and Mesman J. (forthcoming). Taking resilience beyond the science of surprise: contingency, complexity and practice. In: A. Hommels, J. Mesman and W. Bijker, eds, *The Vulnerability of Technological Culture*. Cambridge, MA: The MIT Press.

Hindmarsh, J. and Pilnick, A. 2002. The tacit order of teamwork: collaboration and embodied conduct in anesthesia. *The Sociological Quarterly*, 43, 139–164.

Iedema, R. and Carroll, K. 2010. Discourse research that intervenes in the quality and safety of care practices. *Discourse and Communication*, 4, 68–86.

Iedema, R., Merrick, E. Rajbhandari, D. Gardo, A., Stirling, A. and Herkes, R. 2009. Viewing the taken-for-granted from under a different aspect: a video-based method in pursuit of patient safety. *International Journal of Multiple Research Approaches*, 3, 290–301.

Iedema, R., Mesman, J. and Carroll, K. (forthcoming). *New Perspectives on Clinical Practice Improvement*. Oxford: Radcliffe.

Kohn L. T., Corrigan, J. M. and Donaldson, M. S. (Eds) 1999. *To Err is Human. Building a Safer Health System*. Institute of Medicine. Washington, DC: National Academic Press.

Law, J. 1994. *Organizing Modernity*. Oxford: Blackwell.

Lock, M., Young, A. Cambrosio, A. and Harwood, A. (Eds) 2000. *Living and Working with the New Medical Technologies: Intersections of Inquiry*. Cambridge: Cambridge University Press.

Lomax, H. and Casey, N. 1998. Reordering social life: reflexivity and video methodology. *Sociological Research Online*, 3.

Lynch, M. 1983. Temporal order in laboratory work. In: K. Knorr-Cetina and M. Mulkay, eds, *Science Observed: Perspectives on the Social Studies of Science*. London: Sage, pp. 205–238.

Markussen, R. and Olesen, F. 2007. Rhetorical authority in STS: reflections on a study of IT implementation at a hospital ward. *Science as Culture*. Special Issue: Unpacking 'Intervention' in STS, (16)3, 267– 279.

Mesman, J. 2008. *Uncertainty in Medical Innovation. Experienced Pioneers in Neonatal Care*. Basingstoke: Palgrave Macmillan.

Mesman, J. (2009) The geography of patient safety: a topical analysis of sterility. *Social Science and Medicine*, 69, 1705–1712.

Mesman, J. 2010. Diagnostic work in collaborative practices in neonatal care. In: M. Büscher, D. Goodwin and J. Mesman, eds, *Ethnographies of Diagnostic work: Dimensions of Transformative Practice*. Basingstoke: Palgrave Macmillan, pp. 95–112.

Mesman, J. (forthcoming a) Moving in with care: about patient safety as spatial achievement. *Space and Culture*, special issue (accepted for publication).

Mesman, J. (forthcoming b) The relocation of vulnerability in critical care medicine. In: A. Hommels, J. Mesman and W. Bijker, eds, *The Vulnerability of Technological Culture*. Cambridge, MA: The MIT Press.

Owen C., Wackers, G. and Béguin, P. (Eds) 2009. *Risky Work Environments. Reappraising Human Work With-In Fallible Systems*. Aldershot: Ashgate.

Reason, J. 1990. *Human Error*. Cambridge: Cambridge University Press.

Schmidt, K. and Bannon, L. 1992. Taking CSCW seriously: supporting articulation work. *Computer Supported Cooperative Work*, (1), 7–40.

Strauss, A. 1985. Work and the division of labour. *The Sociological Quarterly*, 26, 1–19.

Suchman, L. 1987. *Plans And Situated Action. The Problem Of Human–Machine Communication*. Cambridge: Cambridge University Press.

Suchman, L. 1996. Supporting articulation work. In R. Kling, ed., *Computerization and Controversy: Value Conflicts and Social Choices*. New York: Academic Press, pp. 407–423.

Suchman, L. 2000. Embodied practices of engineering work. *Mind, Culture, and Activity*, 7, 4–18.

Summerton, J. and Berner, B. (Eds) 2003. *Constructing Risk and Safety in Technological Practice*. London: Routledge.

Vincent, C. 2006. *Patient Safety*. London: Churchill Livingstone/Elsevier.

Wilde de, R. 2000. Innovating innovation: a contribution to the philosophy of the future. Keynote address at Policy Agendas for Sustainable Technological Innovation. London, December 2000.

Woods, D. and Hollnagel, E. 2006. Prologue: resilience engineering concepts. In: E. Hollnagel, D. D. Woods and N. Leveson, eds, *Resilience Engineering: Concepts and Precepts*. Aldershot: Ashgate, pp. 1–16.

Xiao, Y., Seagull, J., Mackenzie, C. and Klein, K 2004. Adaptive leadership in trauma resuscitation teams: a grounded theory approach to video analysis. *Cognition, Technology, Work*, 6, 158–164.

PART 3
Technology

Chapter 5

Deviantly Innovative:
When Risking Patient Safety is the Right
Thing To Do

Emma Rowley

Medical devices are ubiquitous in the delivery of modern day health care (Small 2004, Ward and Clarkson 2004). The UK National Health Service (NHS) is the largest customer of medical devices in the world (Faulkner 2009), with 'many thousands of items used each and every day by health care providers and patients' (MHRA 2007). A medical device can be something as small as a pair of contact lenses or swab, through to a hospital bed or wheelchair, or something more complex and high-tech, such as a magnetic resonance imaging scanner. All have to be fit for purpose before they can be utilized safely within the health care setting.

Increasing attention is given to patient safety and minimizing the risk and frequency of iatrogenic harm. However, in contrast to the attention given to more visible patient safety risks, such as medication errors, patient misidentification or patient accidents (Chassin and Becher 2002, Dean et al. 2002, Taxis and Barber 2003, Cousins et al. 2005), the threats linked to the use of medical devices appear almost negligible. Small (2004: 368) argues that the 'role of devices in medical harms and hazards has lagged behind advances in other areas of safety concerns', whilst Ward and Clarkson (2004: 18) suggest that 'although the scale of errors with medical devices is less clear than that with medical errors in general, the limited evidence that does exist indicates that such errors are also a noteworthy problem'. For example, the most recent data from the UK's National Patient Safety Agency's National Reporting and Learning System (2011) shows that just 35,223 of the 1,157,380 incidents reported about care received in acute NHS Trusts between July 2009–June 2010 were linked to the use of a medical device. In contrast, medication errors accounted for approximately three-and-a-half times as many reported incidents (N = 123,795).

This chapter explores the use of medical devices in relation to patient safety, and in particular, their *misuse*. It outlines how the on-the-ground practicalities and complexities of delivering patient care can influence the decision to misuse medical devices, or indeed use them in innovative ways. It applies an interpretive social science lens to critically examine the reasons for these behaviours with the aim of drawing out and exploring the wider socio-cultural context. The arguments made are based on qualitative data collected in an exploratory study of the reuse of single-use medical devices in the English NHS (see Dingwall et al. 2007).

What do we Know about Medical Devices and Patient Safety?

Whilst some medical device errors are just that, errors and mistakes, it is impossible to examine patient safety without also engaging in a critical analysis of the nature of 'deviancy' and wrongdoing in relation to the use of medical devices. From the examples below, we can see the kind of harm that results from the misuse of medical devices.

> In 2001, 9-year-old Tony Clowes fell of his bicycle and severed a finger. He was taken to Broomfield Hospital (Essex, UK) where he underwent a simple procedure to have his finger sewn back on. However, Tony suffered irreversible cerebral anoxia – oxygen starvation of the brain, and died. The investigation into Tony's death found that part of the anaesthetic breathing circuit had been unwrapped prior to use, contrary to the manufacturer's recommendations. The device had become blocked by the cap from an IV giving set, thus occluding the oxygen supply, leading to the hypoxia. Both the cap that blocked the device and the device itself were made of non-translucent plastic, meaning that the blockage was not visible.
>
> *The Telegraph* (2001), Department of Health (2004), *BBC News* (2006)

> In 2000, Alan Brant had a benign lump in his throat removed at St Peter's Hospital (Surrey, UK). However, he later received a malignant diagnosis and had most of his oesophagus, the top of his stomach and his spleen removed. At a subsequent consultation, Mr Brant was told that he had been misdiagnosed and did not in fact have cancer. The misdiagnosis was blamed on a contaminated pair of biopsy forceps, which had been used to transfer his tissue samples to a pathology slide.
>
> *Daily Mail* (2005), Meikle (2005)

> In 2002, 24 patients at Middlesbrough General Hospital (North Yorkshire, UK) were placed at risk of developing variant Creutzfeld–Jakob Disease (vCJD) due to the contamination of surgical instruments used in their neurosurgical procedures. The instruments had been used in the surgery of an elderly woman, who had presented with headaches and memory loss. When all routine causes of these symptoms had been considered, a brain tissue biopsy was sent to the UK CJD surveillance unit, and a diagnosis of vCJD was finally made. However, in the time between the sample being taken and the results received, the instrumentation had been used in a number of other cases, rather than being

quarantined and later destroyed (as UK guidelines for equipment used on CJD/ vCJD patients demand). As a consequence, 24 patients were subjected to the risk of acquiring vCJD from contaminated equipment.

British Medical Journal (2002), Kirkup (2002)

These cases illustrate the harm that can be done to patients when rules about the use of medical devices are not followed. However, this chapter questions whether breaking the rules *always* results in patient harm. It considers if creating hard and fast rules – rules that should never ever be broken – is the only way of addressing patient safety when using medical devices. By utilizing social science arguments about the nature of mistakes to examine the misuse of medical devices, these questions will be answered and further probe a topic that is critical to the patient safety movement.

Although it is vital to use devices safely, it is also important to consider when breaking rules, so-called 'deviant behaviour', is the only safe and reasonable action to follow. Some health care innovations while created for safety reasons, actually lead to greater patient harm. Likewise, although the majority of medical devices are fit for practice, some, whilst technically 'safe', may help to create errors and risks.

By investigating actual instances in which breaking patient safety rules and conventions might result in improved patient safety outcomes, this chapter asks whether the misuse of medical devices is wrong and constitutes misconduct and deviancy, or might differently be recognized as innovative behaviour and boundary pushing, which leads to the development of surgical science. In addressing these issues, the chapter explores whether errors are always errors, or alternatively, might be understood as examples of what I have chosen to call *deviantly innovative* behaviour. For an action to be classed as deviantly innovative, it must be contrary to the device regulations governing its usage, but is done of the best of reasons – because it enables better care to be provided to the patient, and is therefore the right thing to do.

In the classic text *Limits to Medicine: Medical Nemesis*, Illich (1976) suggests that the medical profession presents a major threat to the health and well-being of the patient. The orthodox safety position is dependent upon the normative assumption that risking the patient's safety is inherently wrong. Moreover, any practitioner knowingly threatening the well-being of their patient is viewed as deviant and morally deficient. This is perhaps best summed up by the statement 'first do no harm', popularly attributed to Hippocrates and his assertion that 'as to diseases, make a habit of two things – to help, or at least do no harm' (Duma 1971: 1258). However, the question that is rarely asked is what is regarded as 'harm'. Focusing on data examining practitioners' rationales for their use medical devices, and in particular, their use of single-use devices, I argue that on occasions it is advantageous for the patient if the practitioner 'breaks' the safety rules in place. In some instances, contravening patient safety regulations may actually protect the patient from greater harm.

More often than not, errors are reported because they have a visible, and sometimes an immediate adverse outcome, such as a medication reaction, a fall, the wrong patient being brought into the operating theatre and, although thankfully rare, a patient fatality. Linking an error and adverse outcome with medical devices can be far more difficult, and consequently, this might explain why fewer incidents are reported. Tracing a post-operative infection to the use of a particular medical device is prohibitively difficult; not only could the actual device have been one of a number of the same item used during the surgical procedure, but it could have been cleaned and sterilized, or discarded prior to the infection developing, and would therefore not be easily traced. Likewise, the practitioner might work around a lack of equipment – or 'accommodate' to use Waring et al.'s (2007) terminology, and continue with the operation, by using an alternative piece of instrumentation. Consequently, Baker et al. (2002: 95) propose that the device errors reported form the 'tip of an iceberg and that many more cases occur that are simply not recognized'.

Single-use Devices

Within the medical device family sits a particular interesting and safety-relevant sub-category of products: single-use devices. As their name suggests, single-use devices should be used once and then discarded. Their *raison d'être* is the prevention of health care-acquired infection and cross-contamination. Single-use devices were introduced into routine surgical practice following awareness that steam and chemical sterilization and decontamination processes were ineffective at removing all microbial and protein or prion-based materials from surgical and anaesthetic instruments (Descôteaux et al. 1995, Will 2003, Baxter et al. 2005).

Historically, the main concern with contaminated medical devices has been the risk of Creutzfeld–Jakob Disease (CJD) and blood-borne diseases such as HIV/Aids and hepatitis (Nielson et al. 1980, Tibbs 1995, Parker and Day 2000). Evidence of iatrogenic transmission of CJD first emerged in the 1950s, when concerns were raised about the possibility that contaminated surgical instruments might infect patients. These were reiterated in the 1970s following iatrogenic cross-infection stemming from the use of cadaveric corneas during transplantation. However, it was not until the iatrogenic transmission of variant Creutzfeld–Jakob disease (vCJD) from one neurosurgical patient to another, and the discovery of prion protein in the appendix of a patient who subsequently developed vCJD, that attention was given to the possibility of the medically induced transmission of the disease (Kirkup 2002, Donaldson 2006).

Single-use devices were designed and introduced with the aim of protecting patients from contamination and cross-infection. However, in recent years, there has been a growing level of concern that some single-use devices might be being reused. A UK survey reported that 10 per cent of responding hospitals admitted reuse of single-use devices (Patients Association 2002). Worldwide, to the reuse of single-use devices appears to be even more widespread. Collignon et al.'s (1996, 2003) surveys of Australian hospitals found that 38 per cent of hospitals were reusing single-use devices, and while another 20 per cent were no longer doing so, they had done within the previous twelve months. In the USA, reprocessing of single-use devices is a frequent activity (Favero 2001).

Drawing on data collected from a study commissioned by the UK's Patient Safety Research Programme to investigate the patterns of reuse in the UK (Dingwall et al. 2007), a potentially more worrying phenomenon became evident (Rowley and Dingwall 2007). Specifically, we found that single-use devices might not provide the patient safety solution as desired in policies. Rather they might actually be harming patient in other ways. Some single-use devices, for instance, were perceived by clinicians to be of such poor quality that they were not fit for purpose or use. Moreover, some practitioners went so far as to suggest that the risk of harm to the patient was greater if they used the single-use device than if the patient had been exposed to a piece of equipment that might have been contaminated or infected with blood or tissue residue remaining from a previous usage. By opting to use the reusable equipment, practitioners behaved *deviantly*, rejecting the guidance governing the device usage, and utilizing equipment that although could theoretically infect a patient, would not bend, break or flex and cause trauma to their body. The remainder of this chapter explores this process and the reasons why it occurs

The Study

A purposive sampling strategy was chosen to ensure the experiences of using single-use devices in a range of hospitals were collected. Sample characteristics included location (urban/rural), geography (Strategic Health Authority boundaries), hospital size (measured by bed numbers) and Healthcare Commission star rating. The final sample compromised of 13 hospitals, which were spread across 8 NHS Trusts and 3 Strategic Health Authorities. All appropriate ethical and governance clearances were received prior to the commencement of data collection.

Theatre managers, theatre nurses, operating department practitioners (ODPs), clinical directors of anaesthesia and sterilization department managers all participated in the interviews. These individuals were selected because they were likely to be involved in the practice of using single-use devices, or were responsible for the management of the theatre/anaesthetic room environment and for stocks of equipment. All interviews were semi-structured and presented comparable questions to all participants; participants were asked to explain their rationales for the local practice of using (and/or reusing) single-use devices and to relate these to current national and local policies and guidelines. They were also asked to talk about the actual use of single-use devices.

In analysing the qualitative interviews, the use of social science helps us to understand that deviancy is a complex concept and that breaking rules may not always be wrong. What might seem at first sight to be an active error (Reason 2000) may be the result of latent failures within the design of devices and regulations, or might not be an error at all, but the outcome of the practitioner's own risk analysis, based upon their clinical knowledge and professional competency. Their activity might break rules and regulations, but they are acting in a manner that they consider to be safe.

Deviantly Innovative?

> In the past, surgical innovation often emerged from unforeseen intra-operative circumstances. The limits between clinical innovation and reckless experimentation were not well defined.

de Leval (2001: 10)

The creation of new forms of knowledge and practice does not occur without testing and pushing at accepted boundaries. New knowledge and practice also shifts expectations of what is considered to be normal or acceptable behaviour, and conversely, what is perceived to be an inappropriate, wrong or deviant act. Although boundary pushing implies the possibility of breakdown and disorder due to 'illegal' behaviour, it is the very nature of science and medicine to test the boundaries of practice, and as de Leval (2001) suggests, to find the limit between clinical innovation and reckless experimentation. Medicine can only develop by continually pushing at its knowledge claims and practice confines.

Clearly, there is an important line between a practitioner being innovative and reckless, but error and harm are not always linked (Layde et al. 2002). A practitioner can do wrong without the patient being hurt or their care being jeopardized. More orthodox patient safety arguments usually see such a scenario as a 'near-miss' (Runciman et al. 1998, Chang et al. 2005). However, by reappraising the situation, we might alternatively see it as an example of the practitioner being 'deviantly innovative'. In the next section of this chapter, data is presented and analysed with the aim of examining when is 'breaking the rules' breaking the rules, and when is 'breaking the rules' making the patient safer. In making this distinction, the chapter will conclude by discussing the issues of recklessness and innovativeness.

Safe Surgery: the 'Deviant' Use of Medical Devices

UK medical device and infection control regulations state that any medical device passing the tonsils should be a single-use device due to the risk of infection and contamination (AAGBI 2002, MHRA 2006). Comparable risks are also present in the appendix and brain. In all other areas of medical practice, the choice of whether to use a single use or reusable device to use is left to the professional discretion of the surgical practitioner. Yet despite the regulations governing practice, the reality of how things actually work or occur at the micro, contextual and everyday level of health care delivery is very different from the static and regimented requirements laid out in legislation at the macro level, which arrives into the clinic from a top-down diktat from Government or hospital management.

In making the decision to break rules and act in an apparently 'deviant' manner, it is important to consider the influence of medical power, medical knowledge and professional status in episodes of deviancy. For example, one theatre manager recalled how a surgeon had a certain set of rules for his own behaviour and practice that was diametrically opposed to the regulations and code of practice that was followed by others:

> We've got a surgeon that has brought a cannula that is a single-use cannula and he's asked us to resterilize it again, arguing 'it's my personal cannula'. I don't care whose it is, you know it's single use and we're not doing it.

> Theatre Manager 5.

The tribalism and the divisive power of professional boundaries and the greater autonomy of surgeons have allowed certain individuals to define their own working practices. The cultural expectation that a surgeon has greater professional status and thus power than, for example, a theatre manager, allows some 'rogue' practitioners to disregard regulations and continue with their practice according to their own rules. For the surgeon described in the data extract, this meant reusing a single-use cannula, thus contravening patient safety regulations. Unlike other accounts that are discussed later in this chapter, no rationalization is given for the reason to reuse the cannula, other than it being 'his own'. Yet unlike the examples seen later in the chapter, this is not an example of innovative behaviour, but of surgical arrogance. Moreover, given that the device cannot be safely resterilized and may therefore be contaminated with another person's blood, it is also an example of recklessness.

Moving away from 'rogue' clinicians and deliberate acts of deviancy, Timmermans and Berg (2003) consider medical devices to be an example of 'technology-in-practice'. The term is used to explain how technology is not a neutral, value-free entity, but is rather negotiated and its meaning defined through its use (Pinch 2010), and as it becomes situated or embedded within the (micro) social context of its use. Similarly, describing the interaction of tasks and technology, Suchman (1987) refers to 'situated actions'. Situated actions describe an activity that may deviate from the intended plan of action once operationalized in the contextual situation. Consequently, a clinician may intend to use a medical device as the manufacturer or regulator intended, only to find this is not possible once in the operating theatre or that the risks of its use are more serious than the risks resulting if another device was used.

This balance of risks echoes some of Beck's (1992) ideas in relation to how society is organized in response to risks, and how we react to perceived hazards through the management and regulation of 'bads' (Hobson-West 2005). However, as a consequence of taking action to counteract the 'bads', new risks are created. Science and technology have long been used to counteract natural risks, with the intention that the intervention will alleviate the risks. However, history shows such activity has often led to new risks. For example, during the late 1950s/early 1960s, Thalidomide was used to ameliorate the symptoms of morning sickness in pregnant women. Whilst it was successful in alleviating the symptoms, it produced unintended side effects: the risk of foetal abnormalities (Møldrup and Morgall 2001). It is in this light that the use of single-use devices should be seen. Single-use devices were introduced to counteract the risk of cross-infection and cross-contamination. However, their use has led to the introduction of different risks.

Consequently, there is a need to examine the situated actions of technology in practice, to establish how practitioners react to both the original and subsequent threats. Webster (2002: 444) outlines how 'technologies are only really successful when they make sense within the existing social relations in which they are to function, suggesting the crucial role played by the translation and even reinvention of technologies into everyday contexts of use'. With this in mind, I now discuss instances in the data where practitioners are using medical devices to respond to risks but where the technology itself creates further risks and so require some translation, moulding or reinvention (so-called deviant innovativeness) to enable them to be used safely.

When talking with practitioners, it became obvious that the single-use gum elastic bougie – a long, slim, malleable device inserted into the patient's trachea and used to guide intubating equipment into place – was neither as effective nor as easy to use as its reusable equivalent. One practitioner described the problem with the single-use bougie and how some clinicians overcame the difficulty with the device by acting in a manner contrary to the guidelines and manufacturer's instructions:

> The gum elastic reusable bougies – they've got memory on them when you bend them, when you bend the tip up by the time you put the laryngoscope in, you want the tip to stay in the position, and with the single-use one, they are just ugh. It's a life-saving bit of equipment … a lot of the anaesthetists still keep the reusables in their briefcase, it's just their little security blanket.
>
> Operating Department Practitioner 2.

Although not directly admitting deviant use of a reusable device, it is clear that the practitioner is questioning the safety and efficacy of single-use bougies. This practitioner's behaviour conforms to the regulations in place: they demonstrate that they ascribe to the goal of the patient safety and the regulated means of achieving this goal, via the use of a single-use device. However, their statement goes on to describe how the safety of the patient is protected by the provision of a fallback, the reusable device kept (deviantly) in the anaesthetist's briefcase as a 'security blanket'. The presence of this 'safety blanket' reinforces the notions of situatedness and technology-in-practice in which safety is seen to be contextually and situational specific (Suchman 1987, Timmermans and Berg 2003). An alternative device is kept for moments of perceived danger and risk, which of course are subjectively recognized and dependant on the practitioners' experience and clinical competency. It is the need to carefully balance safe and reckless behaviour that leads the anaesthetist to use the 'safe' single-use device. However, safety is contextually specific; for example, if the patient gets into ventilation difficulties, then the anaesthetist may consider the only safe solution to be the use of the reliable reusable bougie. However, if the patient is not in difficulty, the use of a reusable bougie – which might carry contaminants, is considered reckless. This distinction between (contamination) safety and (ventilation) safety emerged in an interview with an ODP, a member of theatre staff with responsibility for ensuring that the correct equipment is available for surgeons and anaesthetists to use. The ODP was discussing the risks relating to potential contamination verses the risk of ill-functioning equipment:

> If you've got someone that's about to die, then sod the prions, you just use the reusable.

> Operating Department Practitioner 3.

The decision to break the regulations surrounding which device to use was rationalized in terms of keeping a patient alive. Using a reusable device that may have been exposed to prions, which although 'deviant', was perceived to be a safer option than risking the use of a single-use device that may not have functioned effectively or indeed safely.

The practice of using a reusable device opposed to a single-use device is at the same time both deviant and innovative. Using a reusable device, rather than a single-use device as per the guidelines and regulations, deviates from standard practice and the expectation that a single-use device would be used. According to the rules, it is an example of unacceptable deviant behaviour. However, it is questionable whether the activity would result in a suboptimal outcome, and thus the deviancy might be condoned. Given practitioners concerns about the safety of some single-use devices, the risks presented by the (deviant) use of a reusable device may be more acceptable with regard to the safety of the patient. Practitioners were acting deviantly in order that a greater chance of maintaining patient safety was possible.

Some time after the single-use devices study had concluded, an email arrived in my inbox from an anaesthetist practising in the United States. The anaesthetist agreed with the assessment that some single-use devices were dangerous and risked patient safety (Rowley and Dingwall 2007), and elaborated upon their own practice. They wrote how:

> The most difficult anaesthesia airway management item to find a suitable single-patient-use replacement is the bougie. I must admit that there really isn't anything quite like a [reusable] high-quality gum elastic Eschmann stylet. Since these are typically used only for more difficult intubations, perhaps a more salient question is whether the reusable product should be used as a single-use item? The expense (approximately US$80) is certainly not extravagant, especially when one considers the many other disposable items used for a surgical case, e.g. skin staplers at approximately US$40 each.
>
> US Anaesthetist.

This extract describes an episode of deviant innovativeness. The anaesthetist's account implies that they ascribe to the goal of patient safety, but in order to meet it, must take alternative – deviant – action. Opposed to using a reusable piece of equipment and placing the patient at risk of cross-contamination, they admit to using a reusable piece of equipment as a single-use device, regardless of the greater cost involved in its purchase and disposal. According to Vaughan (1999: 291)

> decisions to violate have been explained by the amoral calculations hypothesis, a form of rational choice theory: Confronted with blocked access to legitimate means to organizational goals, decision-makers will calculate the costs and benefits of using illegitimate means; if benefits outweigh the costs, actors will violate.

The previous three data extracts do not demonstrate any suggestion of amorality or recklessness on behalf of the practitioners. Rather, they detail their attempts to reach a rational, informed decision. For example, the extract from the American anaesthetist reflected their awareness of the risk presented to the safety of the patient by the use of a single-use device, and their considered decision to use a reusable device, albeit as a single-use device. A similar account was given with regards to a piece of surgical equipment:

> We do have some problems as certain instruments have problems with decontamination afterwards. In particular, I'm thinking of orthopaedic sets, and I know that there is a cannulated screwdriver which we use which is designed to be multiple use and cleaned, which the sterilization department claim they cannot do so, and therefore we have been using in single usage. That's a bit of a

problem, as it's just putting a single screw in, and I think it costs in the order of £200 per go, and we dispose of these.

Theatre Manager 6.

In attempting to rationalize the negotiation between practice, risk and patient safety, this practitioner reports how the shortcomings of the medical device were managed. By using a reusable device as a single-use device, the practitioner is showing the greater importance given to patient safety compared to the financial implications of the decision to dispose of a reusable device after only one usage. Whilst this latter action is deviant, and potentially reckless in that it 'wastes' resources, it is also an example of deviantly innovative behaviour. It is breaking the rules to protect the patient from greater harm. Again, what becomes apparent is the situated management of the risk.

Vaughan (1999) argues that routine nonconformity is a normal by-product of techno-scientific work. Given the situatedness of medical decisions, being able to react in a nonconformist manner is critical and protects both the patient and the wider health care system from risk. Star (1995) points out that ad hoc strategies, knowledge and actions can assist an organization to 'keep going' at times of uncertainty. Contravening social rules and acting in a deviantly innovative manner can result in an uncertain situation becoming certain.

Such patterning of deviantly innovative behaviour is neither new nor unique. Off-label usage of medicines and medical devices – usage that falls outside of their licensed and regulated use – continues to occur (Boos 2003). For example, a medication might be used to treat a different patient cohort than the drug was designed for, given in a different dosage, or used in the treatment of an altogether different disease/illness than anticipated by the manufacturers. Data suggests that medical devices are no different, and are used for off-label practice. A theatre manager reported one surgeon's actions in using a medical device in a manner contrary to which it was designed for:

> We've got a surgeon that does thyroidectomics and as part of that he will use a pressure bag that fits around fluid bags and actually pressures the fluid in. Now he'll use that pressure bag inflated to put behind a patient's neck. That's not what it's licensed for, but it does the job thank you very much.

Theatre Manager 5.

The off-label use of medical devices converts disorder into order and is an example of reactive behaviour, whereby the practitioner responds to the situation and context in which the (mis)use/non-legislated use occurs. Here, the theatre manager appears to be implying that the surgeon may have been acting in a rogue manner, commenting 'that's not what it's licensed for, but it does the job thank you very much'. This remark alludes to the greater power and professional status of the surgeon in being able to determine which equipment he is going to use for the procedure. Seen in a different light however, the theatre nurse can be seen as agreeing with the surgeon's decision (which we can only presume was based on his clinical experience and balancing of risks). Whilst the action of using the pressure bag in an off-label manner is deviant, and has not been risk-assessed, it is innovative in that it allows the procedure to go ahead without delay.

Maisel (2004: 300) considers off-label use of medicines and medical devices to be 'part of practice of medicine and reflects the execution of medical judgment'. For Kessler et al. (2004), off-label use is a form of medical experimentation, but importantly it is not considered to be reckless, as it is experientially informed and relies on knowledge, skill and clinical familiarity. Although this type of behaviour is clinically informed, by acting in a manner contravening rules and regulations, the opportunity for errors to occur is presented. Whilst using medical devices off-label enables surgical practitioners to 'get the job done' and convert disorder into order, it presents a threat to patient safety. Over time, the off-label use of medical devices becomes normalized, routinized and accepted, and the 'deviant' practice becomes the standard practice, despite the device not being certified as safe for use in such a manner. Moreover, as such behaviour is dependent on skills, expertize and knowledge, it is likely that the potential risks of harm are much greater if practitioners with less experience are also allowed to make these decisions.

Social theorists and more recently, patient safety advocates, recognize that routine nonconformity results in mistakes, misconduct and disaster (West 2000, Quick 2006). Whilst patient safety research has investigated the causes of why and how things go wrong, there has been little academic attempt to apply a theoretical explanation to the phenomenon. At the heart of the argument that this chapter makes about patient safety is the balance or negotiation between breaking rules, protecting the patient and what is recognized as deviancy or wrongdoing. Vaughan (1999: 286) discusses the sociology of mistakes, and points to the 'processes that neutralize or normalize certain kinds of mistakes, so that people in the workplace see them as routine and non-remarkable'. Vaughan's work is a valuable addition to patient safety research because it provides a theoretical explanation of why errors can repeatedly occur, despite examination, recommendation and identification of learning opportunities to prevent future disasters and incidents. Vaughan (1999: 273) defines deviancy as 'an event, activity or circumstance ... that deviates from the formal design goals and normative standards or expectations, either in the fact of its occurrence or in its consequences, and produces a suboptimal outcome'. If mistakes are left unacknowledged and untreated, they become normalized, routinized and (sub)consciously accepted. They may threaten social cohesion and social stability, and ultimately result in disaster. In terms of patient safety, if mistakes are left unacknowledged and untreated, they also become normalized and accepted as routine, and a critical incident has the opportunity to ensue, as depicted by the holes or gaps in Reason's (2000) 'Swiss cheese' model.

Vaughan (1999, 2005) argues that as a result of the normalization of deviancy, the inevitability of errors is overlooked, whilst the errors themselves are tolerated. Changes in behaviours or norms become accepted, and what was once considered deviant becomes endured, and subsequently identified as normal practice. However, although activity becomes normalized, it is still contingent upon its context. Therefore, the actions perceived by some as deviant and vice-versa, as acceptable, are not always so for others (Merton 1957). They could be reconfigured and reclassified as forms of innovative behaviour or recklessness. Such a shift in conception enables the boundaries of 'right' and 'wrong' to be tested and expanded. There is a risk however, that by concentrating on first-order thinking like the actions described in this chapter, whereby individuals are personally altering their behaviour to counteract a failing device, that the opportunity to improve patient safety at a wider level is overlooked. Practitioners who are using medical devices in a deviantly innovative manner, while protecting patients, are denying the opportunity for broader public awareness of the problems that exist with these devices. This means that the deficiencies of some medical devices cannot be changed for the better. It seems therefore that the danger here is that if the second-order thinking is denied then the problem will only grow, as it cannot be solved by individual practitioners accommodating and working around weaknesses in the design and functionality of medical devices.

Conclusion

The data extracts discussed in this chapter have purposely been selected to highlight examples of practitioners conforming to regulations regarding medical device usage and patient safety, acting innovatively in accepting the goal of patient safety but choosing alternative means in which to achieve the objective, thus being deviantly innovative, and lastly acting deviantly and recklessly. The following discussion is based on the assumption that the culturally agreed goal is the safety of the patient, whilst the institutionally legitimated means of meeting this goal is the correct (as sanctioned in the national regulations) use of medical devices.

When practitioners were reported to have acted deviantly, the rationales for their behaviour relied on explanations linked to cultural and normative assumptions and stereotypes regarding negative surgical reputations. For example, because the 'deviant' practitioner was a surgeon, they could 'get away' with breaching regulations and practice guidelines. Such a justification suggests that the greater power and professional status of practitioners is important when making the decision to use a device incorrectly, whilst other (lower-status) practitioners are unable to prevent the behaviour from continuing or to chastise the practitioner for their actions.

The majority of the data extracts discussed in this chapter demonstrate some level of safety conformity. Practitioners demonstrated that they accepted the culturally ascribed goals of patient safety and the institutionalized means of achieving this goal (the correct, regulated method of using each medical device). However, whilst the goal of patient safety was internalized, in many of the cases that initially appear to demonstrate conformist behaviour, the means of realizing the goal were ultimately rejected. Displaying what I have called 'deviantly innovative' behaviour, practitioners decided to use equipment that they believed to provide the safest option. For example, the US anaesthetist and the theatre manager who recalled the use of a reusable cannulated screwdriver, both reported how they chose to meet the goal of patient safety by using reusable devices albeit as single-use devices. This action enables patients to have clean equipment used in their care, whilst at the same time enabling practitioners to be confident that they were using safe equipment that was fit for practice.

Returning to one of my opening questions – can patient safety be managed by hard and fast rules? The examples and discussion within this chapter go some way to saying no, it cannot. Whilst rules clearly have a place, there should be some flexibility to enable them to overcome unforeseen risks and consequences that arise within the contextual setting.

All of the data extracts presented in this chapter reinforce Collins' (1992) suggestion that in conditions of uncertainty, actors convert disorder to order. Medical equipment that was considered to risk or threaten the safety of the patient, despite being approved for practice, was rejected in order that patient safety could be guaranteed. According to Vaughan's (1999) arguments, such action constitutes deviancy as it contravenes culturally ascribed means of achieving the desired goal. However, as the practitioners' rationales testify, they considered that their so-called deviant actions offered a better patient safety solution. They were acting in a deviantly innovative manner.

So, to return to my second question – is rule-breaking wrong and reckless, or is rule-breaking an example of innovativeness? The evidence-based arguments made have demonstrated that rule-breaking is situationally specific. Some rule-breaking is inherently wrong (for example, the surgeon and his 'own cannula'). Actions can be reckless and the consequences can be devastating. Yet at other times, clinicians need the freedom to operate in the safest possible manner, and this can mean that they need to break the rules. Waring et al. (2007) suggest that clinicians subconsciously tolerate, accommodate or innovate against risk, and that key to these actions is the autonomous professional discretion of the practitioners. They found that professionals made 'an implicit decision about risk, whereby the risks of introducing unorthodox practice was balanced against the overall risks to patient health and "getting the job done"' (Waring et al. 2007: 5). Such an argument is confirmed in the data discussed in this chapter, whereby practitioners relied on their clinical expertise and knowledge to recognize and act upon the threat that certain medical devices presented to the safety of the patient.

Waring et al. (2007) echo Vaughan (1999), and warn that as practitioners tolerate, accommodate and innovate to address the shortcomings of the health care system, these behaviours become customary, and in turn become a haven for risk. In relation to the use of medical devices, the normalization of the deviant act of using a non-single use item creates the risk that the threat of cross-contamination and infection will eventually be overlooked, allowing safety lessons to go unheeded, and possibly resulting in a patient safety disaster. It also creates a situation where the shortcomings of single-use devices are not addressed, as practitioners do not report their problems, but conceal them with their use of alternative equipment.

The central problem with the normalization of deviancy is what Hall (2003: 241) refers to as 'the very pragmatic notion of "acceptable" deviance'. Whilst being deviantly innovative may push the development of medical science, or enable the job 'to be done', it can introduce new threats to health care, and reintroduce old ones. Vaughan (2005) warns that by accepting deviation, practitioners are on a slippery slope to disaster. A theoretical understanding on deviancy allows us to see the structural or macro understanding of error and the normalization of deviancy. In contrast, a micro approach enables the inadequacies of macro-level theorizing to be observed, and allows us to see how patient safety is negotiated within the specific and fluid context in which safety is being sought. Single-use devices were established for valid patient safety reasons; that they are not used in some cases is also for valid patient safety rationales. Clinicians are being deviantly innovative in order to protect the patient. If the founding rule of medicine is 'first do no harm', then clinicians must have medical devices that are safe to use. Rules and regulations should not be allowed to override or obscure clinical common sense. Patient safety needs to move beyond structural thinking and more standardized examples of system-based learning (Leape et al. 1998, Nieva and Sorra 2003, Waring 2005), to instead focus on the micro-environment in which clinicians practice and make split-second, situated patient safety decisions. If we are to learn anything from the risk society thesis, it should be this: by reacting to risks, we create new risks. Regulations that are created to manage risks should not be able to restrict practice to such an extent that the new risks cannot themselves be controlled.

It is not the intention that the take-home message of this chapter should be 'ban all regulation'. Medical device regulations are needed, and do protect patients (and staff) from harm. However, in some cases – in contexts in which the situation is uncertain – the presence of regulations should not be allowed to overrule clinical experience and clinical common sense. Although practitioners need to exercise greater awareness of the potential for errors with routinized non-conformity, sometimes behaving in a deviantly innovative manner might protect the patient from a harm that may present itself when the practitioner acts in a conformist manner.

Acknowledgements

The data discussed in this chapter is drawn from Dingwall et al. (2007). *Patient Safety: Reuse of Single Use Devices*, and was funded by the Department of Health's Patient Safety Research Portfolio (ref: PS022), 2004–2006. The report is available to download at: http://pcpoh.bham.ac.uk/publichealth/psrp/Publication_PS022. htm.

References

AAGBI (Association of Anaesthetists of Great Britain and Ireland). 2002. *Infection Control in Anaesthesia*. London: AAGBI.

Baker, N. Tweedale, C. and Ellis, C.J. 2002. Adverse events with medical devices may go unreported. *British Medical Journal*, 325, 905.

Baxter, H.C., Campbell, G.A., Whittaker, A.G., Jones, A.C., Aitken, A.A., Simpson, A.H., Casey, M., Bountiff, L., Gibbard, L. and Baxter, R.L. 2005. Elimination of transmissible spongiform encephalopathy infectivity and decontamination of surgical instruments by using radio-frequency gas-plasma treatment. *Journal of General Virology*, 86(8), 2392–2399.

BBC News. 2006. NHS trust fined over boy's death. 31 January 2006. http://news. bbc.co.uk/1/hi/england/essex/4667738.stm, accessed 14 June 2006.

Beck, U. 1992. *Risk Society: Towards A New Modernity*. London: Sage.

Boos, J. 2003. Off label use – label off use? *Annals of Oncology*, 14, 1–5.

British Medical Journal – News. 2002. Inquiry into handling of CJD alert welcomed. *British Medical Journal*, 325, 1055.

Chang, A., Schyve, P.M., Croteau, R.J., O'Leary, D.S. and Loeb, J.M. 2005. The JCAHO patient safety event taxonomy: a standardized terminology and classification schema for near misses and adverse events. *International Journal for Quality in Health Care*, 17(2), 95–105.

Chassin, M.R. and Becher, E.C. 2002. The wrong patient. *Annals of Internal Medicine*, 136(11), 826–833.

Collignon, P.J., Graham, E. and Dreimanis, D.E. 1996. Reuse in sterile sites of single-use medical devices: how common is this in Australia? *Medical Journal of Australia*, 164(9), 533–536.

Collignon, P.J., Dreimanis, D.E. and Beckingham, W.D. 2003. Reuse of single-use medical devices in sterile sites: how often does this still occur in Australia? *Medical Journal of Australia*, 179(2), 115–116.

Collins, H.M. 1992. *Changing Order*. Chicago, IL: Chicago University Press.

Cousins, D.H., Sabatier, B., Begue, D., Schmitt, C. and Hoppe-Tichy, T. 2005. Medication errors in intravenous drug preparation and administration: a multicentre audit in the UK, Germany and France. *Quaity and Safety in Health Care*, 14(3), 190–195.

Daily Mail, The. 2005. £192,000 for man falsely told he had cancer. *Daily Mail*, 12 January. http://www.dailymail.co.uk/health/article-333816/192-000-man-falsely-told-cancer.html#ixzz1HJu4rqcE, accessed 17 November 2007.

De Leval, M. 2001. From art to science: a fairy tale? The future of academic surgery. *Annals of Thoracic Surgery*, 72, 9–12.

Dean, B., Schachter, M., Vincent, C. and Barber, N. 2002. Prescribing errors in hospital inpatients: their incidence and clinical significance. *Quality and Safety in Health Care*, 11, 340–344.

Department of Health. 2004. *Protecting the Breathing Circuit in Anaesthesia. Report to the Chief Medical Officer of an Expert Group on Blocked Anaesthetic Tubing*. London: Department of Health. http://www.dh.gov.uk/ assetRoot/04/08/18/26/04081826.pdf, accessed 31 October 2004.

Descôteaux, J.G., Poulin, E.C., Julien, M. and Guidoin, R. 1995. Residual organic debris on processed surgical instruments. *Association of Perioperative Registered Nurses Journal*, 62(3), 23–30.

Dingwall, R., Rowley, E., Currie, G., Aikenhead, A., Wilson, J., Sharples, S. and Norris, B. 2007. *Patient Safety: The Reuse Of Single Use Medical Devices. Final Report to the Patient Safety Research Programme*. http://pcpoh.bham. ac.uk/publichealth/psrp/Publication_PS022.htm, accessed 1 November 2007.

Donaldson, L. 2006. *Protecting the Public: Creutzfeldt–Jakob Disease*. London: Department of Health. http://www.dh.gov.uk/en/Aboutus/ MinistersandDepartmentLeaders/ChiefMedicalOfficer/Features/ FeaturesBrowsableDocument/DH_4102718, accessed 22 April 2006.

Duma, R.J. 1971. First of all do no harm. *New England Journal of Medicine*, 285, 1258–1259.

Faulkner, A. 2009. *Medical Technology into Healthcare and Society: A Sociology Of Devices, Innovation And Governance*. Basingstoke: Palgrave Macmillan.

Favero, M.S. 2001. Requiem for reuse of single-use devices in US hospitals. *Infection Control and Hospital Epidemiology*, 22, 539–541.

Hall, J.L. 2003. Columbia and Challenger: organizational failure at NASA. *Space Policy*, 19, 239–247.

Hobson-West P. 2005. *Understanding vaccination resistance in the UK: radicals, reformists and the discourses of risk, trust and science*. Ph.D. thesis, University of Nottingham.

Illich, N. 1976. *Limits To Medicine: Medical Nemesis – The Expropriation Of Health*. London: Boyars.

Kessler, L., Ramsey, S.D., Tunis, S. and Sullivan, S.D. 2004. Clinical use of medical devices in the 'Bermuda triangle'. *Health Affairs*, 23(1), 200–207.

Kirkup B. 2002. *Incident Arising in October 2002 from a Patient with Creutzfeldt– Jakob Disease in Middlesbrough. Report Of The Incident*. London: Department of Health

Layde, P.M., Maas, L.A., Teret, S.P., Brasel, K.J., Kuhn, E.M., Mercy, J.A. and Hargarten, S.W. 2002. Patient safety efforts should focus on medical injuries. *Journal of the American Medical Association*, 287, 1993–1997.

Leape, L.L., Woods, D.D., Hatlie, M.J., Kizer, K.W., Schroeder, S.A. and Lundberg, G.S. 1998. Promoting patient safety by preventing medical error. *Journal of the American Medical Association*, 280(16), 1444–1447.

Maisel, M.H. 2004. Medical device regulation: an introduction for the practicing physician. *Annals of Internal Medicine*, 140, 296–302.

MHRA (Medicines and Healthcare Products Regulatory Agency). 2006. *Device Bulletin: Single Use Medical Devices – Implications and Consequences of Reuse DB2006(04)*. http://www.mhra.gov.uk/home/idcplg?IdcService=SS_ GET_PAGE&useSecondary=true&ssDocName=CON2024995&ssTargetNod eId=572, accessed 23 March 2006.

MHRA (Medicines and Healthcare Products Regulatory Agency). 2007. *What we Regulate: Devices*. http://www.mhra.gov.uk/home/idcplg?IdcService=SS_ GET_PAGE&nodeId=78, accessed 3 October 2007.

Meikle, J. 2005. Needless throat op left man 'devastated'. *The Guardian*, 12 January. http://www.guardian.co.uk/society/2005/jan/12/2?INTCMP=SRCH, accessed 17 February 2005.

Merton, R.K. 1957. *Social Theory and Social Structure*. New York: Free Press.

Møldrup, C. and Morgall, J.M. 2001. Risk society – reconsidered via a drug context. *Health Risk and Society*, 3(1), 59–74.

National Patient Safety Agency. 2011. *NRLS Quarterly Data Workbook Up To September 2010, Reference 1313*. London: National Patient Safety Agency. http://www.nrls.npsa.nhs.uk, accessed 22 March 2011.

Nielson, E., Jacobsen, J.B., Stokke, D.B., Brinklov, M.M. and Christenson, K.N. 1980. Cross-infection from contaminated anaesthetic equipment. *Anaesthesia*, 35, 703–708.

Nieva, V.F. and Sorra, J. 2003. Safety culture assessment: a tool for improving patient safety in health care organizations. *Quality and Safety in Health Care*, 12, ii17– ii23.

Parker, M.R.J. and Day, C.J.E. 2000. Visible and occult blood contamination of laryngeal mask airways and trachael tubes used in adult anaesthesia. *Anaesthesia*, 55, 367–390.

Patients Association. 2002. *Infection Control And Medical Device Decontamination: A Survey Of Strategic Health Authorities*. London: Patients Association.

Pinch, T. 2010. On making infrastructure visible: putting the non-humans to rights. *Cambridge Journal of Economics*, 34(1), 77–89.

Quick, O. 2006. Outing medical errors: questions of trust and responsibility. *Medical Law Review*, 14, 22–43.

Reason, J. 2000. Human error: models and management. *British Medical Journal*, 320(7237), 768–770.

Rowley, E. and Dingwall, R. 2007. The use of single use devices in anaesthesia: balancing the risks to patient safety. *Anaesthesia*, 62(6), 569–574.

Runciman, W.B., Helps, S.C., Sexton, E.J. and Malpass, A. 1998. A classification for incidents and accidents in the health-care system. *Journal of Quality in Clinical Practice*, 18(3), 199–211.

Small, S.D. 2004. Medical device – associated safety and risk: surveillance and stratagems. *Journal of the American Medical Association*, 291(3), 367–370.

Star, S.L. 1995. *Ecologies Of Knowledge: Work And Politics In Science And Technology*. Albany: State University of New York Press.

Suchman, L.A. 1987. *Plans And Situated Actions: The Problem Of Human–Machine Communication.* Cambridge: Cambridge University Press.

Taxis, K. and Barber, N. 2003. Causes of intravenous medication errors: an ethnographic study. *Quality and Safety in Health Care,* 12, 343–347.

Telegraph, The 2001. How could someone end my little boy's life? *The Telegraph,* 19 August. http://www.telegraph.co.uk/news/uknews/1337916/How-could-someone-end-my-little-boys-life.html, accessed 17 November 2007.

Tibbs, C.J. 1995. Methods of transmission of Hepatitis C. *Journal of Viral Hepatitis,* 2(3), 113–119.

Timmermans, S. and Berg, M. 2003. The practice of medical technology. *Sociology of Health and Illness,* 25(3), 97–114.

Vaughan, D. 1999. The dark side of organizations: mistake, misconduct and disaster. *Annual Review of Sociology,* 25, 271–305.

Vaughan, D. 2005. Organizational rituals of risk and error. In: B. Hutter B and M. Power, eds, *Organizational Encounters With Risk.* Cambridge: Cambridge University Press, pp. 33–66.

Ward, J.R. and Clarkson, J.P. 2004. An analysis of medical-device related errors: prevalence and possible solutions. *Journal of Medical Engineering and Technology,* 28(1), 2–21.

Waring, J., Harrison, S. and McDonald, R. 2007. A culture of safety? Ritualistic behaviours in the operating theatre. *Journal of Health Services Research and Policy,* 12(1; supplement), 3–9.

Waring, J.J. 2005. Beyond blame: cultural barriers to medical incident reporting. *Social Science and Medicine,* 60(9), 1927–1935.

Webster, A. 2002. Innovative health technologies and the social: redefining health, medicine and the body. *Current Sociology,* 50(3), 443–457.

West, E. 2000. Organizational sources of safety and danger: sociological contributions to the study of adverse events. *Quality in Health Care,* 9, 120–126.

Will, R.G. 2003. Acquired prion disease: iatrogenic CJD, variant CJD, Kuru. *British Medical Bulletin,* 66, 255–265.

Chapter 6

The Precarious Gap between Information Technology and Patient Safety: Lessons from Medication Systems

Habibollah Pirnejad and Roland Bal

Despite the advances in organizing safe practice in health care, medical errors are still common and costly. Health Information Technology (HIT) has recently received much attention from health care authorities as a great potentiality to improve patient safety. Some studies, however, have reported on the generation of new types of medical errors due to Information Technology (IT) applications in health care. Therefore, understanding the mechanisms through which IT can cause or compound errors in medical practice is a basic step towards the safe application of HIT in health care. In this chapter, based on empirical evidence from our own field studies and those of others, we analyse the conditions in which working with information systems can result in error or increases the risk of error in medical practice. Three main mechanisms are discussed here: interoperability problems, dissociation between virtual and real practices, and workflow impediments. Each mechanism is described and supplemented with examples from health care practice. While we argue that these mechanisms are fundamental issues to IT use, some of their effects on patient safety can be remedied by situated reflexivities on their consequences.

> Prescribing medication is not easy. It is almost impossible to know all possible combinations of drugs and which combinations are harmful. It is also almost impossible to know the precise composition of all drugs to avoid sensitivity reactions in your patients. This means it is highly risky to prescribe medication without automated systems that signal possible contra-indications and drug-drug interactions. For doctors, using these systems is possible for almost twenty years now but still in practice many drugs are prescribed without the use of such systems. This is imposing unnecessary risk ... and is no longer justifiable ... Therefore I announce that as of 1 January 2012 all prescribers should use computerized physician order entry (CPOE) systems.[1]

van der Wal 2010.

---

[1]   All quotes from the Dutch have been translated into English by the authors.

Cries like this one from the Chief Inspector of health care in the Netherlands are by now common in the health care field. Errors in medical practice are challenging health care providers and organizations to provide safer care for patients. Despite advances in the way care practices are organized and delivered, medical errors are still prevalent and can lead to serious side effects (Institute of Medicine 1999, Committee on the Quality of Health Care in America 2001, Barber et al. 2003). The HARM study in the Netherlands, for example, found that 5.6 per cent of all acute hospital admissions are related to medication errors, of which almost half (16,000 per year in total) could have been prevented (Leendertse et al. 2008).

There are many reasons for this. However, one thing is very clear, the more health care practice grows in terms of the involved parties, the more it grows complex and error prone. Organizing and coordinating different care providers working on the same group of patients is a challenge for modern health care practice. So far, many approaches have been applied in order to reduce the possibility of errors and to improve patient safety. None of these approaches have attracted the attention from health care authorities to the extent of that seen with HIT. There are many places in health care where HIT can potentially reduce errors and improve quality of care and patient safety (van Bemmel and Musen 1997, Bates et al. 2001, Bates and Gawande 2003): it has been considered a central component of many health care reforms and has been invested in heavily. For example, the UK has invested £12.3 billion on its national IT project (NPfit) (Brennan 2005), and President Obama has recently committed to invest a total of $US 50 billion over five years 'to move the U.S. health care system to broad adoption of standards-based electronic health information systems, including electronic health records'.[2]

The improving effects of HIT on patient safety have been a principal motivation for health care organizations to adopt these solutions (Committee on the Quality of Health Care in America 2001). However, despite their great potentiality, the evidence concerning their contribution to patient safety is not very solid. Some recent studies have reported the ways these systems compounded medical errors (Ash et al 2004, Koppel et al. 2005). Many of these HIT side effects have been hidden or hard to recognize by *in vitro* studies and through ordinary evaluation methods. They reveal themselves when HIT interacted in real life care practice and via in-depth qualitative studies of the implementation sites (Pirnejad et al. 2009). In this chapter, we evaluate the effect of HIT on patient safety and try to illuminate important mechanisms through which these systems may function in a counterproductive manner. This way, we hope to identify lessons to be learned in promoting patient safety in the design and application of HIT.

In this chapter, we elaborate upon the mechanisms being activated as the result of socio-technical interactions of health care environment with HIT and present these mainly in the form of silent or latent errors in the course of care practices. More specifically, three interconnected mechanisms are of concern which come into effect through working with HIT. They are: interoperability impeding,

---

2   http://www.barackobama.com/pdf/issues/HealthCareFullPlan.pdf.

dissociation of virtual and real practices, and workflow impeding. Some of these mechanisms, we argue, are fundamental to IT use and can be very well explained by concepts drawn from the social science of technology and safety. The analysis presented here is supplemented by evidence from our extensive study on HIT and patient safety as well as from studies by others. In the conclusion we return to the question of how such analyses can be used to improve patient safety.

Studying Technologies in Practice

There is a long tradition of studies in science and technology studies (STS) challenging mainstream conceptions of the relationship between technology and society. Rather than conceptualizing technology as a tool to solve societal problems, empirical work in this tradition has shown that it is more productive to view this relation as a form of co-construction or co-shaping (Bijker and Law 1992; Hackett et al. 2008). Technologies are not developed autonomously and then have an 'impact' on society (such as technological determinism would have it), nor do societal processes determine the development of technology. Rather, specific technologies are developed alongside specific societal interactions and processes and the two co-constitute each other.

This work departs in significant ways from the Rogerian notion of technology development and diffusion, which is central to much health care policy and research (Greenhalgh et al. 2004). In the first place, technology, in the STS version, does not have inherent properties such as usability or relative advantage. Such characteristics, which are central to a Rogerian take on technology, are instead analysed as accomplishments of the specific practices in which technology is put to use. Technologies have to be 'domesticated' in order for them to work and in this domestication process, both the practice and the technology change. For example, in a study on Louis Pasteur, Latour has shown that in order for vaccination to become successful, French society needed to be changed according to the laboratory conditions in which the vaccination could work. Similarly, however, vaccines themselves had to be moulded in order for them to become usable in such diverse practices as French rural and urban settings (Latour 1988, Callon et al. 2009).

Such research on the practice of technology (Timmermans and Berg 2003) also points to the crucial role for the users of technologies. Rather than merely being 'innovators' or 'laggards', as diffusion theory might have them, users actively shape the technologies they encounter. Whereas technologies often contain 'scripts' on the ways in which they are supposed to be used (think of your own struggles with photocopiers or what it was like to learn to drive a car or ride a bicycle), users are proficient in de- and re-scripting technologies in order to make them 'fit' into their own practices (Akrich 1992, Oudshoorn and Pinch 2003). This also implies that the implementation of technologies – if implementation is taken to mean the direct application of a technology as it was developed and meant to be used – is a rare, if not impossible event.

Thirdly, and closely related to the 'scriptedness' of technologies, STS work has shown that technologies are not neutral tools, but rather reinforce or change existing social relations. Information technologies, for example, not only often presuppose a temporal order of activities, but are also built on social relations between, say, medical specialists, nurses and patients. While they coordinate work between those different social actors, they also presume specific roles of each of them (Berg 1999). Technologies, in this sense, are actors in their own right (Latour 1992).

This alternative take on the relation between technology and society is consequential for the role information technologies can play in relation to patient safety. As evidenced with the quote from van der Wal with which we started this chapter, information technologies are often seen as tools to improve patient safety if only their obstinate users start using them in the ways they are supposed to be used. However, from an STS perspective there can be no such straightforward relation between technologies and use. Rather, we have to focus on the practices in which information technologies are embedded, the ways in which they are used, how they shape social relations and are reshaped in turn. This also means that there can be no straightforward relationship between the use of technologies and patient safety. As technologies get moulded in practice, their specific properties also get shaped, changing the ways in which they were supposed to work. This can either take the form of 'working around' the technologies, or adapting them to the specific needs of users (as Rowley shows in Chapter 5). As a consequence of such domestication processes, the initial supposed effects of the use of technology for patient safety get distorted. This finding is corroborated by many studies on industrial accidents (Jasanoff 1994, Vaughan 1996, Hutter and Power 2005).

In order to study the consequences of the use of information technologies in health care for patient safety, it is thus necessary to give a detailed account of the practices associated with their use. We therefore proceed with a detailed analysis of information technologies in use, with a special focus on medication systems.

Interoperability as a Practical Accomplishment

For care providers to coordinate throughout a collaborative care process, they have to successfully communicate information. Successful communication, however, is not simply information exchange between the communicators. For a successful communication, care providers have to gain mutual understanding over the exchanged information, as they have to use the exchanged information to proceed with patient care (Pirnejad et al. 2008b).

Interoperability is defined as 'the ability of parties, either human or machine, to exchange data or information' (Mead 2006, 73). In medical informatics, the term interoperability is often used to describe the connection between information systems. An extended application of interoperability can be used to imply care providers mutual intelligibility over the exchanged information, either through direct interaction with each other, for example, through face-to-face communication, or through interaction with patient care information systems, such as paper-based or HIT systems (Pirnejad et al. 2008b). With such a broadened definition, the concept of interoperability can provide a framework for evaluating sociotechnical interactions with information systems and for understanding the work that is needed to transfer information from one community into a shared arena. Interoperability can, however, not be supposed to exist a priori, but is something which needs to be established in specific practices.

Interoperability problems in HIT happen mainly because of problems in information flow between care providers (Pirnejad et al. 2009). This happens, for example, because an information system supports a highly collaborative care process only partially. It can also happen if care providers have to work with different but not integrated or partially integrated information systems within a collaborative care process. In either case, interoperability problems can either directly or indirectly lead to error in care providers' practices.

Contexts of Information Production and Use

Without doubt, information systems improve the physical appearance (for example, the legibility) of exchanged information in comparison to paper-based systems. This improvement, however, does not necessarily improve mutual intelligibility of care providers concerning the exchanged information (Pirnejad et al. 2008b). In an evaluation of a computerized physician order entry (CPOE) system at Erasmus Medical Center (Pirnejad et al. 2009), we found that the system significantly improved legibility and layout of prescriptions in comparison to those received within the paper-based system. However, electronic prescriptions caused nurses to make mistakes in reading and executing the orders. The prescription printouts were small and contained many (and sometimes unnecessary) information with no indicator to emphasize the important items, and this made nurses susceptible to mistakes. This kind of error was especially common when nurses had to read and complete many prescriptions quickly, for example during busy shifts, and when a patient was transferred from one ward to another with a lot of prescriptions that had to be reprinted in the new ward. Many of those errors were normally discovered and corrected during the evening or night shifts when paper-based medication administration records were double-checked against patients' medicine cabinet and their current medication lists printed from the system. However, other mistakes might not come to light for some time and patients might receive wrong medications or incorrect doses for quite a while. For instance, one Head Nurse stated that:

> During the night shifts, nurses distribute 24 hours worth of patients' medications into their medication cabinets. After 24 hours the cabinets have to be empty, but sometimes they are not. Then we have to check and see what happened and what

the reason was. Sometimes you discover that some of the prescription labels are missing from the patient administration reference, or they are put in the wrong patient records. But sometimes you have no idea what exactly has happened.

Head Nurse.

The orderly world of computers is not easily translated into messy health care practices. The activity outlined above in the nursing ward is quite similar to what happens at other wards. Consider for example Balka and colleagues' study of the introduction of an automated drug dispenser (ADD) in a nursing ward (Balka et al. 2007). While the ADD is part of an orderly medication chain in the hospital, connecting the pharmacy to the wards, the practice of medication distribution in the ward creates a disorderly parallel world. For instance, whereas the ADD presupposes that nurses hand out medication at specific time intervals, patient routines at the ward prohibit this from happening in all cases. As a result, medication piles up just next to the ADD. The 'inherent safety' that was presupposed in the ADD in this way is unmade in practice. Or, in other words, the orderly world of the ADD creates its own disorder right next to it and the two – order and disorder – constitute each other (Berg 1998).

The reality that most communication through HIT is normally asynchronous adds to the messiness of putting HIT to use. Within time-intensive care processes, asynchronous communication can hamper mutual intelligibility of care providers and as a result their, collaboration. In our study of the CPOE system, nurses for example were receiving prescriptions asynchronously and failed to communicate their feedback and comments to physicians easily and in a timely fashion. Thus for instance, when physicians, especially junior physicians and residents, made a mistake, informing them about these mistakes became difficult after the CPOE system was implemented. The only way for nurses to correct these mistakes was to pick up the printed prescriptions and then find the prescribing physician, either directly or on the telephone, something which was time-consuming for already busy nursing staff (Pirnejad et al. 2008b). In asynchronous communication, there is also the possibility that putting information into the information system is misunderstood as a complete communication process and the necessary checks on mutual intelligibility are neglected. For example, we observed that sometimes physicians forgot to inform nurses that they had issued new prescriptions in the CPOE system. Under such conditions, there were considerable opportunities for the prescription printouts to be lost in nursing stations, or to be neglected especially if nurses were busy and away from the printer's location.

Information is a context-dependent entity, and its meaning will change if it is used within different contexts or for different purposes (Berg and Goorman 1999). For interoperability of care providers to be achieved, the information must be put in the right context. This has two important consequences. First, a good understanding of the context in which information is produced and used is necessary for care providers to perform an interoperable communication. Secondly, if information transaction is supposed to connect care providers' practices across different boundaries, connecting working contexts should precede the information transaction. If, for example, primary and secondary care providers are supposed to work on the same set of patient data, the related care processes at both sides have to be aligned and integrated first (Pirnejad et al. 2008a, Pirnejad 2009). In a study of a communication network between primary and secondary health care (Pirnejad et al. 2008a), we found many interoperability problems despite the existence of an almost ideal technical condition for information exchange. In this project, the same information and coding systems were used on both sides of the communication network. Nevertheless, many communication errors occurred that hampered interoperability of care providers upon the exchanged information. For care providers at the hospital, for example, a considerable amount of information received from primary care was nonsense, something that could potentially lead to errors in their practice. In addition, it was found that community pharmacists were registering information in their information system in a way which was intelligible considering their working context, but which could produce problems for care providers at the secondary health care level who were unaware of this information context; whilst at the same time, GPs frequently registered 'the status is OK' indicating that patients' current medication was updated and there was no need for any adjustment. Such information only became mutually intelligible when care providers spent extra effort in solving such ambiguities. Such problems are not unique to this particular situation; in a project on electronic referrals in another region in the Netherlands we observed similar occasions of interoperability problems stemming from the idiosyncratic use of information systems (Bal et al. 2007, Bal and Mastboom 2007).

Working Around Health Information Technologies

Interoperability problems within a collaborative health care process can restrict synchronization and coordination between care providers and as a result undermine work consistency and integration. The work process in such conditions will be disrupted and proceeding from one stage of care into another becomes difficult for care providers. To compensate for interoperability problems and to improve the disrupted care process, care providers devise informal rules and procedures in working with health information technologies. That is, they 'work around' the system to get the work done. These work arounds are considered necessary for care processes which without them will grind to a halt. The work arounds, however, can be unsafe for patients and pose considerable risk of error to care providers' practice (Pirnejad et al. 2009). For example, we observed that because logging in and out into the system was considered time-consuming, physicians normally postponed sending prescription orders to nurses until they could do them all at once. Although this solved the physicians' problem to some extent, they caused a lot of problems for nurses as they were not getting authorized prescriptions in time. Nurses, as a result, did not wait for physicians' prescriptions and began their medication work based on the notes they took during medical rounds. Moreover, they accepted verbal instructions from physicians but wrote them down on paper-based forms both for legal purposes and to remind physicians to enter them into the system later (Pirnejad et al. 2009). Those work arounds were not safe compensating strategies: they increased the risk of error in nurses' and physicians' practice.

While work arounds have been shown to be problematic in many instances (Wynne 1988, Ash et al. 2004) they are necessary parts of working with (health information) technologies, more particularly in dealing with the lack of fit between the scripts embedded in technologies and the practices in which they are supposed to work. Work arounds are thus not an expression of failing technologies but are an integral part of working with technologies in practice. Safety problems with work arounds occur in those instances where the presumed behaviour of users goes against the safety guards that are embedded in the technologies; in the case of our CPOE system this happens because the system works from the presumption that all medication prescriptions have to be authorized by medical specialists, whilst at the same time the system prohibits this from happening during the round. Prescriptions therefore get delayed, causing the nurses to work from their notes, which creates the possibility for errors to occur. While refining the technology, in this case for example by using PDAs during the round, might prevent these errors to occur, this might also create new needs for work arounds.

Virtual–real Dissociations

Information systems contain a model of the processes which they are designed to support. This model determines what steps in the care process have to be done by who, when, where, and in what sequence. This conceptual model can be called the virtual practice in comparison to the real practice which it corresponds to. Many errors in working with information systems occur because connections between the virtual and the real worlds become problematic in patient care. Dissociation between virtual–real practices can happen for many reasons and can cause error in patient care both directly and indirectly.

Direct Effect

One of the great advantages of using HITs is that patient data can be stored and saved for use along the patient trajectory. Problems may occur however during the time the virtual and real versions of patient care are coupled, especially at the time the patient is admitted. A patient, for example, may get a wrong digital ID (or barcode) at the admission time which assigns a wrong virtual care process to the patient. Consequently, wrong laboratory tests may be requested, wrong decisions upon the patient may be made, or wrong medication may be started for the patient

(Hakimzada et al. 2008). Likewise, a faulty system entry can cause the right data to be assigned to the wrong patient. For example, because of a keyboard entry mistake one patient may have two different identification numbers and their data might be split over two completely separate sets of records (Bradley et al. 2006, Hakimzada et al. 2008).

Indirect Effect

Health information technologies are necessarily standardized but have to be used in sometimes extremely variable health care practices. Therefore, there is a great possibility that the care processes in real life may not match well to the process designed into a system. As a result, virtual processes might, either intentionally by the users or automatically by the system, create dissociations between virtual and real practices. A barcode medication administration which has a strict timing for the medication administration may, for example, halt the process at hand because a nurse exceeds the time expected by the system (Patterson et al. 2002, Koppel et al. 2008). Such dissociations can cost time, increase workloads and lead to error-prone practices.

When case-critical information regarding a patients' care trajectory (for example, when and where a patient has to receive their care) is changed in real practice but is not updated in the system, virtual–real practice dissociation will happen. For example, when a patient is moved from one room or one ward into another, or is changed from one medical condition into another (for example from post anesthesia to normal ward condition) and information systems are not updated in this regard, virtual–real practice dissociation can cause errors in patient care. Medications, as a result, may be sent to a wrong patient, or seized medications in the system may not be reactivated for quite a while after an operation (Koppel et al. 2005). Moreover, the necessary speed of real care processes can cause the requirements of linking virtual and real practices to be overridden. For example, in emergency situations, life-saving measures (such as the administration of medications) normally precede information system updates. This delayed update of information systems, although unavoidable, can cause errors to health care practices. In such post hoc updates there is a significant possibility of data loss and that some parts of the information will never be registered into the information systems (Pirnejad et al. 2008b). Even in 'normal' situations, complete medical records are the exception rather than the rule, as much information is considered to be redundant for actual care processes where the patient is an additional source of information, whether through asking or through other types of bodily examination (Berg 1999). Sharing of information is thus never complete.

Workflow Impeding

Working with information systems may conflict or hamper the flow of health care work. Depending on the severity of this conflict and to the reaction of care providers, workflow problems can lead to errors in health care providers' practice or they can be compensated either with extra work of care providers and/or by devising informal ways of working with the system (work arounds). Although devised work arounds can improve the flow of care process, many of them can pose risks to patient safety (Koppel et al. 2008, Vogelsmeier et al. 2008). The existing conflict may create negative emotions towards a system, and in turn decrease the cognitive ability of care providers to handle complex situations thereby resulting in increased possibility of error(s) in their practice. The conflict between workflow and working with information systems can be due to many reasons. For example, as discussed previously, if working with information systems causes communication problems between care providers, this will break their workflow.

A simplified and stepwise workflow process modeled into an information system may only correspond to care providers' routine work. Thus, it will conflict with deviation from routine which is sometimes necessary for the management of collective and ad hoc organized health care practice (Gorman et al. 2003, Niazkhani et al. 2010). At Erasmus Medical Center, for example, we observed that unless physicians completed the prescription stage of the medication process by entering prescriptions into the CPOE system, nurses could not order non-stock medications from the pharmacy department. While before the implementation of the system nurses had enough authority to do so, the system did not allow them to proceed with their medication work unless physicians completed the prescription work. For good reasons, however, physicians delayed entering their medication into the system and this caused a lot of inconvenience and extra work for nurses who needed to keep the medication process running smoothly. For example, if a necessary medication was ordered late, nurses had to go to the pharmacy department directly or had to call pharmacists (and explain the reason of the delay) in order to make sure that the medication was going to be supplied in a timely fashion. To compensate for this, nurses in different wards gradually adopted different informal and sometimes unsafe strategies. For example, they were giving medications to patients out of other patients' medication stocks kept at the ward, or they borrowed the medication from a neighbourhood ward.

Likewise, the stepwise workflow process with an information system may increase the number of necessary steps for an action. For example, to modify or change an order within the CPOE system, physicians have to cancel the previous order first and then create a new one with the necessary changes in the system. This increases the risk that old orders fail to be discontinued and such failures have been reported as a potential source of error in evaluation studies (Koppel et al. 2005).

Like many CPOE and other information systems in use in health care, the specific system in use on the wards we studied reproduced the hierarchy between doctors and nurses and presupposed a handbook version of the medication process. Whereas this may in theory be good for patient safety, in practice the underlying scripts of the CPOE system caused many problems. Working with information systems may, and does, interfere with care activities. Care work is performed within a dynamic situation where care providers, patients, care resources and information sources are dynamic and moving around (Bardram and Bossen 2005). If the design of an information system cannot afford the necessary level of mobility in care work, it will hamper the flow of work and as a result will lead to compensative reactions of care providers to repair the hampered processes. For example, working with a barcode medication administration system requires scanning the patients' barcode wristband before giving the medication to a patient. However, studies reported that this can interfere with patients' activity. Thus, nurses' work will come to a halt and the system may drop the task at hand if they cannot find patients in their beds at the time of medication administration. To compensate, nurses administered medication without scanning the patients' barcode. This, however, increases the chance of giving the wrong medication to patients (Koppel et al. 2008). As another example, in our field research, we observed that physicians were either memorizing or taking small notes about changes they were intended to make on patients' medications because the CPOE system was not accessible at the patients' bedside. This way of working with short notes and abstract information increased the cognitive load of physicians and as a result they sometimes forgot the details or made mistakes in their practice.

Working with information systems has a threat of undermining the professional ability and clinical insight of care providers. As clinicians get used to organizing and performing their work with information systems gradually, they develop more dependence on these systems and their advice (through alerts) to afford complex care processes (Ash et al. 2007). This runs the risk of error in practice whenever the information system is not available, is down, or has 'crashed'. This becomes more important for new clinicians who do not have experience of working with a backup paper-based system. As one senior attending told us:

> This is a department of gastroenterology. Last weekend, we admitted a patient who was using extensive mediation for her Parkinson disease which are rare medications for our department. The CPOE system was not available because of changing from one version of the program into another which caused some problems in some computers. So, the resident ordered the patient medications on paper and she made a mistake. And the nurse requested the wrong medication from the pharmacy. This [error] happened because the resident was not familiar with the medication and there was no [CPOE] system to help her.
>
> Attending medical specialist.

As health care practice becomes more electronic and technologically based, and because unexpected incidents in information technology are not rare, this overdependence on HIT systems will be a new source of medical error.

Within a collaborative care process, there are many overlaps between the tasks of different professionals. These overlaps help health care professionals to negotiate and connect their work into a whole entity of a collaborative process. If an information system forces a strict level of task authorization, it will also reinforce professional boundaries between care providers. In such a situation, a task or responsibility of one professional may conflict with that of another. For example, we observed that a CPOE system was assigning nurses' tasks or that of pharmacists to the physician with respect to determining the specific route of medication administration (Niazkhani et al. 2010). In this regard, a senior pulmonologist stated that:

> [in the system] if I have 'Dexamethasone', which I [normally] prescribe intravenously or orally. I don't need a complete list. I just need to give it orally or intravenously. The distinction between IV, just IV infusion, IV red, IV white, IV central … [is something that] you don't want to know. It is very specialized [for me].

> Pulmonologist.

There is no doubt that the prescription is the physicians' responsibility; however there are many details concerning the form and administration route of medications which fall in a grey zone of responsibility between nurses, physicians and pharmacists. Physicians normally do not train and do not have enough knowledge to handle this kind of responsibility. Thus, by forcing strict levels of task authorization, information systems can assign tasks of one professional into another, and as a result cause puzzling, knowledge gaps and create the potential for error in practice.

Conclusion

Health information technology is increasingly being called upon to tackle patient safety. Underlying these policies is an understanding that the processes built into information systems will change the health care practices in which they are used in such a way that these will act safely. In this chapter, we have shown that this assumption is wrong. Not only are information technologies reshaped as they are implemented in health care practices, they can also become causes of error in themselves. In this chapter, we presented three error-contributing mechanisms that come into effect following the implementation and use of information technologies in health care: interoperability problems, dissociation between virtual and real practices and workflow impediments. We illustrated these mechanisms with excerpts taken from our observations of medication information systems in use and with the work of our colleagues, who have analysed similar practices in widely differing health care systems. We believe these error-causing mechanisms to be fundamental to information technology use. Even though specific problems might be corrected – for example, through introducing PDAs for use during medical rounds – such new systems are likely to cause new and unexpected safety problems.

Although this chapter has shown the ways in which information technologies contribute to medical errors, we do not want to argue against the use of information technologies in health care. Such use can and does have many benefits to both safety and efficiency of care. Rather, we argue that analyses as presented in this chapter are on the one hand necessary corrections to overly optimistic policy discourses, and on the other can be used to improve the functioning of these systems in practice. Technology implementation can be conceptualized as an ongoing process that is not finished when the technology is in place, but continues sometimes years on end in which constant (re)adjustments are made to the technology. Reflecting upon these practice adjustments gives much information about the lack of fit between technologies and working practices. In this regard, work arounds can be considered to be ethnographies-in-practice, giving much insight into the moments of tension between practical workflows and technologies, thus functioning as evaluations in practice. Building on such work arounds can lead to innovations in the technology, improving the fit between practices and technologies. Secondly, even when work arounds and other forms of reflection-in-action are used to improve fit, lack of fit will remain and so will other error-prone practices concerning information technologies. Given the complex, dynamic nature of health care work, and given the nature of working with (information) technologies, this is probably inevitable. This entails that focusing on the resilience of health care work remains crucial.

References

Akrich, M. 1992. The description of technical objects. In: *Shaping Technology/ Building Society: Studies in Sociotechnical Change*, edited by W.E. Bijker and J. Law, Cambridge, MA: MIT Press, pp. 205–224.

Ash, J.S., Sittig, D.F., Poon, E.G., Guappone, K., Campbell, E. and Dykstra, R.H. 2007. The extent and importance of unintended consequences related to computerized provider order entry. *Journal of the American Medical Informatics Association* 14 (4):415–423.

Ash, J.S., Berg, M. and Coiera, E. 2004. Some unintended consequences of information technology in health care: the nature of patient care information system-related errors. *Journal of the American Medical Informatics Association* 11 (2):104–112.

Bal, R. and Mastboom, F. 2007. Engaging with technologies in practice: travelling the North-west passage. *Science as Culture* 16 (3):253–266.

Bal, R., Femke R., Mastboom, H. Spiers, F. and Harm Rutten, H. 2007. The product and process of referral. Optimizing GP-specialist communication through ICT. *International Journal of Medical Informatics* 76S (Supplement 1):S28–S34.

Balka, E., Nicki, E., Kahnamoui, N. and Kelsey Nutland, K. 2007. Who is in charge of patient safety? Work practice, work processes and utopian views of automatic drug dispensing systems. *International Journal of Medical Informatics* 76 (Supplement 1):S48–S57.

Barber, N., Rawlins, M. and Dean Franklin, B. 2003. Reducing prescribing error: competence, control and culture. *Quality and Safety in Health Care* 12:i29–i32.

Bardram, J.E., and Bossen, C. 2005. Mobility work: the spatial dimension of collaboration at a hospital. *Computer Supported Cooperative Work* 14 (2):131–160.

Bates, D., Cohen, M. Leape, L. Overhage, M. Shabot, M. and Sheridan, T. 2001. Reducing the frequency of errors in medicine using information technology. *Journal of the American Medical Informatics Association* 8 (4):299–308.

Bates, D.W. and Gawande, A.A. 2003. Improving safety with information technology. *New England Journal of Medicine* 348 (25):2526–2534.

Berg, M. 1998. Order(s) and disorder(s): of protocols and medical practices. In: *Differences in Medicine*, edited by M. Berg and A. Mol. Durham and London: Duke University Press, pp. 226–245.

Berg, M. 1999. Accumulating and coordinating: occasions for information technologies in medical work. *Computer Supported Cooperative Work* 8 (4):373–401.

Berg, M. and Goorman, E. 1999. The contextual nature of medical information. *International Journal of Medical Informatics* 56:51–60.

Bijker, W.E. and Law, J. (eds) 1992. *Shaping Technology/Building Society: Studies in Sociotechnical Change*. Cambridge, MA: MIT Press.

Bradley, V.M., Steltenkamp, C.L. and Hite, K.B. 2006. Evaluation of reported medication errors before and after implementation of computerized practitioner order entry. *Journal of Healthcare Information Management* 20 (4):46–53.

Brennan, S. 2005. *NHS IT Project: the Biggest Computer Programme in the World … Ever!* Oxford: Radcliffe Medical Press.

Callon, M., Pierre, M., Lascoumes, P. and Barthe, Y. 2009. *Acting in an Uncertain World. An Essay on Technical Democracy*. Cambridge, MA: MIT Press.

Committee on the Quality of Health Care in America, Institute of Medicine. 2001. *Crossing the Quality Chasm: A New Health System for the 21st Century*. Washington, DC: National Academy Press.

Gorman, P.N., Lavelle, M.B. and Ash, J.S. 2003. Order creation and communication in health care. *Methods of Information in Medicine* 42 (4):376–384.

Greenhalgh, T., Glenn, T., Robert, F.G., MacFarlane, P.F., Bate, P. and Kyriakidou, O. 2004. Diffusion of innovations in service organizations: systematic review and recommendations. *Milbank Quarterly* 82 (4):581–629.

Hackett, E.J., Amsterdamska, O., Lynch, M. and Wajcman, J. 2008. *The Handbook of Science and Technology Studies*. Cambridge, MA: MIT Press.

Hakimzada, A.F., Green, O.R.A., Sayan, J.O.R., Zhang, J. and Patel., V.L. 2008. The nature and occcurence of registration errors in the emergency department. *International Journal of Medical Informatics* 77 (3):169–175.

Hutter, B and Power, M. (eds) 2005. *Organizational Encounters with Risk*. Cambridge: Cambridge University Press.

Institute of Medicine. 1999. *Too Err is Human: Building a Safer Health System*. Washington, DC: National Academies Press.

Jasanoff, S. (ed.) 1994. *Learning from Disaster: Risk Management after Bhopal*. Philadelphia, PA: University of Pennsylvania Press.

Koppel, R., Metlay, J.P., Cohen, A., Abaluck, B., Localio, R., Kimmel, S.E., and Strom, B.L. 2005. Role of computerized physician order entry systems in facilitating medication errors. *Journal of the American Medical Association* 293 (10): 1197–1203.

Koppel, R., T. Wetterneck, T., Telles, J.L. and Karsh, B-T. 2008. Workarounds to barcode medication administration systems. *Journal of the American Medical Informatics Association* 15 (4):408–423.

Latour, B. 1988. *The Pasteurization of France*. Harvard, MA: Cambridge University Press.

Latour, B. 1992. Where are the missing masses? The sociology of a few mundane artifacts. In: *Shaping Technology/Building Society: Studies in Sociotechnical Change*, edited by W. E. Bijker and J. Law. Cambridge, MA: MIT Press, pp. 225–228.

Leendertse, A., Egberts, A., Stoker, L., van den Bemt, P. and HARM Study Group. 2008. Frequency of and risk factors for preventable medication-related hospital admissions in the Netherlands. *Archives of Internal Medicine* 168 (17):1890–1896.

Mead, C.N. 2006. Data interchange standards in health care IT. Computable semantic interoperability: now possible but still difficult, do we really need a better mousetrap? *Journal of Healthcare Information Management* 20 (1):71–78.

Niazkhani, Z., Pirnejad, H. van der Sijs, A., de Bont, J. and Aarts, J. 2010. Computerized provider order entry system. Does it support the interprofessional medication work? *Methods of Information in Medicine* 49 (1):20–27.

Oudshoon, N. and Pinch, T. (eds) 2003. *How Users Matter: The Co-construction of Users and Technology*. Cambridge MA: MIT Press.

Patterson, E.S., Cook, R.I. and Render, M.L. 2002. Improving patient safety by identifying side effects from introducing bar coding in medication administration. *Journal of the American Medical Informatics Association* 9 (5):540–543.

Pirnejad, H. 2009. Invited commentary. *The Journal of Information Technology in Healthcare* 7 (1):43–45.

Pirnejad, H., Roland, H., Bal, R. and Berg, M. 2008a. Building an inter-organizational communication network and challenges for preserving interoperability. *International Journal of Medical Informatics* 77 (12):818–827.

Pirnejad, H., Zahra, H., Bal, R. and Berg, M. 2008b. Inter-organizational communication in health care. Consideration for standardization and ICT application. *Methods of Information in Medicine* 47 (4):336–345.

Pirnejad, H., Niazkhani, Z., van der Sijs, H., Berg, M. and Bal, R. 2009. Evaluation of the impact of a CPOE system on nurse–physician communication: a mixed method study. *Methods of Information in Medicine* 48 (4):350–360.

Timmermans, S. and Berg, M. 2003. The practice of medical technology. *Sociology of Health & Illness* 25 (3):97–114.

van Bemmel, J.H. and Musen, M.A. 1997. *Handbook of Medical Informatics*. Houten: Bohn Stafleu Van Loghum.

van der Wal, G. 2010. Medicatieveiligheid en elektronische gegevensuitwisseling. Toespraak van de Inspecteur-generaal [Medication safety and electonic data exchange. Speech from the Inspector-general] Paper read at Medicatieveiligheid en ICT, 29 September, Nieuwegein.

Vaughan, D. 1996. *The Challenger Launch Decision: Risky Technology, Culture and Deviance at NASA*. Chicago, IL: The University of Chicago Press.

Vogelsmeier, A.A., Halbesleben, J.R.B. and Scott-Cawiezell, J.R. 2008. Technology implementation and workarounds in the nursing home. *Journal of the American Medical Informatics Association* 15 (4):114–119.

Wynne, B. 1988. Unruly technology. *Social Studies of Science* 18:147–167.

PART 4
Knowledge Sharing

Chapter 7

The Politics of Learning:
The Dilemma for Patient Safety

Justin Waring and Graeme Currie

Learning has become the mantra of health care reform around the world. This is nowhere more evident than in the case of patient safety where health policies argue that if we are to deliver efficient, effective and, importantly, safe care we must learn from past experiences and share our lessons (Institute of Medicine 1999, Department of Health 2000, World Health Organization 2004). It is only through learning that past instances of patient harm, injury or death are not repeated and that innovative and new ways of working are disseminated more widely. In this way, health care organizations become learning organizations.

It is interesting to note that within policy, learning is largely portrayed as a positive activity with beneficial outcomes. Learning is seen as a rational, linear and developmental process involving the acquisition and production of new knowledge around which service improvements can be delivered. This problem-centred view of learning is different from more situated or social models of learning. Moreover, the act of learning is portrayed as being free from bias and as politically neutral. We would argue that questions of power, politics and control are interweaved within the processes of learning (Willis 1977, Lawrence et al. 2005). When such issues are discussed in the context of patient safety this is most evident in relation to the problem of blame, which is said to inhibit learning because prevailing attitudes tend to narrowly lay responsibility for patient harm with those immediately involved rather than the wider system (Reason 1997, Department of Health 2000). It is perhaps because of this blame culture and its detrimental effects on organizational learning that health policies promote learning as largely neutral with positive outcomes, so as not to discourage staff participation and engagement.

This chapter explores how and to what consequence the processes of organizational learning, specifically those associated with improving patient safety, are imbued or characterized by dynamics of organizational power and politics. We do not seek to understand whether staff are simply blamed for reporting, but rather we look more at the micro-sociology world of learning, acknowledging that learning is inherently embedded within a given social, cultural and political context, encompassing specific social interactions and roles, and involving the promulgation of particular values, norms and ideologies. It is necessary to acknowledge, at least, the underlying tensions between health care professionals and service managers that have characterized, even stymied a succession of health care reform agendas

(Light 1995, Flynn 2004, Harrison 2004). When located within this wider context, patient safety reforms are confronted with a challenge that goes beyond how best to introduce to new risk management systems, but instead touches upon more deeply embedded political fault lines in the organization of health care service. When asking critical questions about the patient safety movement, analysis must therefore consider these shifting tectonics of organizational politics and power. This involves considering how learning systems may function as a mechanism of authority and power, through the control of information and through informing organizational and occupational change, as well as being attentive to the potential resistance to these systems.

    The chapter begins with an overview of the forms of organizational learning being developed and implemented within health care systems around the world, including Australia, Canada, Malaysia, the UK and the USA (World Health Organisation 2004). It is argued that the broad approach reflects the models of learning and risk regulation found in other industries and economic sectors, most notably aviation and petrochemicals. In an attempt to mimic these seemingly highly reliable organisations, health policies have drawn narrowly upon the advances made in these other sectors, copying key components and techniques but sometimes neglecting the nuanced realities of health care. With specific reference to the UK National Health Service (NHS), detailed consideration is given to the National Reporting and Learning System. After reviewing the study approach, the chapter presents an empirical account of how issues of organizational politics feature within and shape these processes of learning.

Learning Around Patient Safety: the Mainstream Approach

Over the last ten or so years, health policies have consistently questioned the capacity for health care organizations to effectively learn the lessons for patient safety (Institute of Medicine 1999, Department of Health 2000, World Health Organization 2004). As discussed in the introduction to this collection, the growing body of international evidence not only reveals the worrying level of patient morbidity and mortality brought about by our health care systems, but in doing so it reveals the deficiencies and inadequacies of our existing regulatory and managerial systems to learn effectively from these experiences. The UK report *An Organization with a Memory* showed that health care providers rely upon a myriad of loosely linked regulatory, managerial and legal systems, yet these have consistently failed to promote a systematic approach to learning that ensures past mistakes are not repeated (Department of Health 2000). The general consensus of opinion is that existing systems to monitor and assure clinical quality and risk are typically disparate, isolated within particular occupational enclaves, characterized by sectional bias and not sufficiently robust in promoting widespread learning (Walshe 1999). It has been repeatedly shown, for example, that a complex and embedded range of informal and collegial practices have a powerful role in hoarding knowledge related to the quality and safety of clinical care (Freidson 1970, Rosenthal 1995, Kennedy 2001, Smith 2004). This was powerfully demonstrated, for example, by a series of high-profile scandals in the UK where established regulatory systems were shown to protect the interests of the profession above and beyond those of patients (Kennedy 2001, Smith 2004).

With mounting evidence of clinical risk and the apparent inadequacy of existing systems to learn effectively about the endemic threats to patient safety, health policies have sought to bring about a fundamental shift in how we think about, respond to and learn from clinical risks. Industries such as aviation, nuclear energy and petrochemicals have been hailed as examples of high reliability because of their proven safety record and capacity to learn from safety events. Safety experts have extolled the ways in which such industries manage and learn from risk and safety events (Reason 1997, Reason and Hobbs 2003). In doing so, they have sought to translate these ideas and techniques and apply them within the health care sector. As discussed in the introduction to this collection, this has included a significant re-conceptualization of safety drawn from ergonomics and human factors. This has also involved formulating systems that, as in these other industries, engender the sharing of knowledge about safety events and stimulate learning. Although international variations are evident, health care providers around the world are endeavouring to develop more robust systems of organizational learning. These are largely concerned with establishing procedures, such as incident reporting, to routinely capture information about safety events, and techniques such as root cause analysis to inform their investigation (see Mengis and Nicolini, Chapter 9 this volume).

For the UK NHS, this is found in the National Reporting and Learning System (NRLS) (National Patient Safety Agency 2003). In common with systems of learning found in other health care systems, and also other industries, the NRLS can be seen as comprising three core stages. The first involves establishing systems and procedures to routinely and effectively capture information about the adverse events and near misses that threaten patient safety. As with other industries, a dedicated incident reporting system has been implemented across the NHS with the expectation that all health care providers, professionals and even patients or their families will share their experiences of potential or actual patient harm. The completion of incident reports typically involves describing the nature of the event, including who was involved, where and when it took place, what form (or type) did the incident take, what was the impact on the patients health, what were the contributory factors, and what remedial action was taken. These incidents are to be reported, initially, to local service leaders responsible for patient safety, and then nationally to the NPSA. The idea is that this information will inform learning within local service providers as well as at a service-wide national level. Of significance, this process is envisaged as being geared towards positive organizational learning, as opposed to negative individual blame.

The second stage involves analysing and interrogating this information to identify the underlying causal factors and relative significance of the event. The

NPSA has invested considerable resources and time in guiding and supporting these analytical and investigation activities, including a nationwide campaign of training for local risk managers. Here, it is anticipated that incidents will undergo an initial process of risk stratification that is geared towards determining the relative status and significance of the incident, followed by more structured and systematic investigation in the form of root cause analysis. Common to all approaches is a desire to understand the contributory and causal factors that produced the given event so as to inform organizational change and safety improvement.

The third stage encourages service leaders, and the NPSA at the national level, to utilize this information to initiate safety improvements. Specifically through understanding more about how upstream factors intersect with and shape clinical practice it becomes possible to devise new ways of working to limit the reoccurrence of risk. The prevailing literature highlights a range of possible areas for making change, from the organization and management of resources, to interprofessional working and the ergonomics of equipment design. This involves trying to make clinical practice less error-prone through introducing, often formulaic, guidelines and protocols that stipulate how clinicians should undertake tasks that are known to be high risk.

Policies recognize that the success of such systems is contingent upon fostering cultural change, especially the introduction of a safety culture than encourages openness and reporting, and therefore counters a blame culture (Department of Health 2000). However, we also need to understand more about how health care professionals experience and engage with these new processes if we are to be confident that they are capable of delivering the level of learning expected in health policy and required for service improvement.

The Study

This chapter draws upon the findings of an ethnographic study of the introduction of the NRLS within two NHS hospitals undertaken between 2000 and 2005. The research involved prolonged periods of direct observation of, and in some instances, participation in the introduction of these new reporting systems. These were largely focused on the work of corporate hospital managers and risk managers, who had responsibility for implementing and managing the new patient safety systems. Participant observations included working alongside members of staff in each hospital risk management department as they processed and filtered reported incidents. Alongside observations, the study involved qualitative semi-structured interviews with managerial and medical representatives. This included a sample of between five–eight clinicians based with five medical and organizational specialties, including acute (internal) medicine, surgery, anaesthetics, geriatrics (care of the elderly) and obstetrics. The interviews followed a thematic guide that explored their prevailing understanding and perceptions of the patient safety problems, their established practices and techniques for addressing safety-related problems, their views about and experiences of the new reporting system, and their preferences for future activities for addressing patient safety. The research findings were analysed to explore how medical professionals interact with the new reporting and learning systems, with a particular view to understanding how this interaction reflected, and perhaps reinforced, underlying tensions between doctors and managers in the UK NHS.

Doctors Interaction with New Learning Systems

Drawing upon empirical observation and interview data in two NHS hospitals, we describe three broad ways doctors engage with these new systems. In doing so, we surface not only the tangible actions and reactions of doctors, but also reveal the underlying cultural assumptions and desires of these professionals about the sharing of information about clinical practice and safety, which in turn brings to the fore not only the underlying cultural barriers to knowledge sharing (Waring 2005, Currie et al. 2008), but also the undercurrents of power and resistance.

Participation

It would be wrong to suggest that all doctors, at all times, do not participate in reporting systems. Although it may appear, as we develop our discussion, that doctors often refrain from procedures that require them to produce evidence of the actual or potential patient harm associated with their practice, we find that many doctors see enormous merit in these new reporting channels, and patient safety activities in general. As we go on to suggest, however, it is often the form and control of these systems that worries doctors, not necessarily the process of documenting and reporting events. Moreover, doctors widely support the idea of new techniques to improve learning around patient safety. Bearing in mind that such views may have been offered in the context of our interviews, the vast majority of our participants claimed the safety and well-being of patients was vital to their work:

> Obviously, the safety of patient care is paramount. It's what we work towards, otherwise we wouldn't be here, would we?

> Doctor.

> I am really happy to get involved with anything that will improve the way we work and help to make the hospital a safer environment for our patients. You see it all the time these days, the patients certainly do with things like MRSA, so we have to do more to make the way we work safer.

> Doctor.

Our discussions with doctors highlighted frequent examples of them completing incident reports in a variety of contexts and in relation to varying types of incidents. To some extent it might be argued that these examples were offered as some form of proof of participation for the research team, and that far from being routine there was often an underlying motive or rationale for reporting that suggested that participation was indeed out of the ordinary, unfamiliar and special:

> I made a report only last week. We had a particular problem within the delivery of surgical instrumentation and I thought to myself this has happened too many times recently. So I wanted to do something and complaining to the theatre staff doesn't seem to get you anywhere so I thought I would try filling an incident report.

Doctor.

Looking across the examples given by doctors it appeared that participation was informed by a number of underlying cultural expectations and assumptions about how work should be organized and a strategic desire to invoke change. For many doctors it was important to report events that were perceived as severe, critical or significant or what they saw as a major, but also irregular threat to patient safety. For example, surgeons often described their work as being high risk and a very real threat to safety, but this was seen as inevitable and therefore only unusual variations in surgical care were seen as significant. This suggests therefore that for some doctors, issues of risk or safety are perceived along some form of spectrum, scale or typology, where certain types of risk are seen as an inevitable 'part of the job'.

It was also clear that the willingness of doctors to report incidents can be motivated by other factors, such as concerns about legal action, the presence of witnesses or pressure from other staff groups. For example, one doctor described a situation where they felt compelled to complete a report because the event had been observed by two nurses who they believed would also report the event. Rather than being motivated by the best interests of the patient or the advancement of learning, reporting was guided by the doctor's desire not to be seen as concealing the truth, as well as to ensure that the nurses' stories of the event were not incorrect or portrayed the doctor in a negative light:

> There was a case about a year ago when a patient was given the wrong medication, it was nothing life-threatening, just a mix-up and the patient was fine in the end, but I reported it because the two nurses were concerned and said a report should be made. So I thought it was right and proper that I fill out a form so that the hospital got the fullest details about what happened from all those present.

Doctor.

Other anecdotal accounts of reporting were also identified that further reveal something important about doctors attitudes towards new patient safety systems. The first can be described as 'superficial participation'. This is when doctors report seemingly trivial and inconsequential events that are perceived as having no direct bearing on the safety of patient care, such as missing stationery, faulty lighting in non-clinical settings and a lack of car parking. These appear to mock the hospitals system through wasting time and resources and could be interpreted as a form of resistance or misbehaviour:

> I often wonder what exactly we are supposed to report. I spent a few days writing up everything I could think of, silly things that really made no difference to the way we worked or the care the patients received. I suppose I was just trying to make a point.

> Doctor.

The second form of participation can be described a 'political participation'. This is when doctors use incident reporting to flag-up issues that align with an existing or ongoing campaign within the hospital. A prominent example related to three surgeons who were petitioning hospital managers for extra resources to purchase new equipment. In this instance, reports were made to reveal problems with existing equipment thereby generating a body of evidence to be used in requesting additional resources. This illustrates the way incident reporting can be used as a lever to support particular arguments or claims within the hospital.

Despite clear evidence of medical reporting, it remained a small proportion of total reported incidents in both hospitals (between 3–8 per cent). Moreover, medical reporting appeared to reflect a wide set of views and assumptions around patient safety. For some, reporting is seen as contributing to learning, but often in extreme or unique situations. In other occasions reporting is undertaken for more strategic reasons, such as to protect professional reputation or to mock managerial efforts. However, the overwhelming view of managers, as recipients, and doctors, as reporters, was that doctors significantly under-report. A large body of evidence describes some of the contextual, cultural and organizational reasons for the lack of medical reporting (Waring 2005, Currie et al. 2008). Whatever the reason, such under-reporting means that the NRLS only receives a limited range of reports and might suffer from significant bias in subsequent risk-management activities, whilst important lessons continue to be lost.

Resistance

Although doctors place enormous value on patient safety and the need for better learning, we found that they held significant reservations about the NRLS and in the main resisted calls for greater reporting. Why then do doctors feel unwilling to share with others knowledge about patient safety? Is this simply a fear of blame or are there other underlying social and cultural reasons for resisting these systems? When talking through these issues it appeared that doctors did not believe the NRLS was the best or most appropriate means of achieving learning and a number of important issues appeared to shape their resistance to this system.

Blame features significantly within health policy as a barrier to learning, and, perhaps unsurprisingly, it features in doctors' justifications for not reporting. It was widely believed that by sharing information doctors could only expect to receive more, rather than less blame from managers and service leaders. As well as managers, a further source of blame was identified with the profession itself. It was felt that increased information about a clinician's safety-related practice could lead colleagues and superiors to question their clinical competence, and perhaps result in disciplinary action or referral to the General Medical Council. For example, one doctor described how incident data could block professional progression because of the old culture of preferment. This might suggest that the desire for cultural change and the fostering of a no-blame culture might not be penetrating front line clinical work:

> I don't care what they say, you just know what is going to happen, they will see your name and they will see the incident and before you know it you are being investigated and held to account. It doesn't matter that they call it no-blame, because the process itself will just equate to being blamed.

Doctor.

One might question, however, whether blame merely provides a convenient explanation for not wanting to report, given the attention in policy? Although many participants talked of colleagues who had been blamed after reporting an incident, there were few specific examples from those we interviewed.

One significant reason for not reporting incidents, which might also explain the enduring concern with blame, was doctors' belief that managers, and indeed outsiders more generally, could not appropriately understand and interpret the clinical details and contexts associated with incidents. This is a long-standing line of reasoning that has reinforced claims to professional autonomy and self-regulation since the mid-1800s (Freidson 1970). However, within the current climate of service rationalization, especially the use of evidence-based medicine and the application of performance management and audit (Harrison and McDonald 2008) such arguments have again risen to the fore of medical resistance to change. This reveals an additional line of resistance, not only towards reporting, but towards health care reforms that extend managerial, or non-medical influence of clinical knowledge and practice. The doctors interviewed in this study overwhelmingly believed that managers working in a centralized risk-management department were not appropriately positioned, experienced or knowledgeable to understand the day-to-day realities of clinical practice and safety, nor were they best positioned to lead the processes of learning and change. Doctors even questioned whether training in the general principles and practices of risk management could really help managers translate and understand the technical clinical information contained within reports given that such training was regarded as abstract and managerial. Doctors scepticism about management was further compounded by a lack of feedback or sustained improvement in the delivery of patient care following the submission of incident reports. Several doctors described how they had received no formal response after reporting and had witnessed no improvements around the problems raised:

> Management could not really comment on the doctor's assessment, the details of history, the details of the examination.

> Doctor.

> The worry is managers don't actually understand medicine. I see things differently, I deal with different things, but management deal with other things, it's all about quality but they can't understand what I do clinically.

> Doctor.

The scepticism about hospital managers appeared to lead doctors to two broad interpretations of the new patient safety systems. The first was that, far from trying to improve the quality and safety, it was seen as another superficial or pointless exercise in data collection. For instance, many doctors saw it as simply another bureaucratic exercise within the NHS, with its associated demands for red tape, form filling and completing meaningless paper trails. The bureaucratic duties and procedures associated with incident reporting were therefore interpreted as antithetical to the ideals of medical practice that are centred on delivering patient care. Although doctors see that more of their work was being subject to bureaucratic rule and paperwork, they believe that learning about the everyday risks of clinical practice was not necessarily achieved through an additional level of form filling:

> It's just collecting data for the sake of it because somebody in management has to tick a box.

> Doctor.

> The work of the risk management is about guards around emergency exits on the stairs, but we haven't seen to the everyday events that are happening.

> Doctor.

What am I going to get out of it, or what is the patient going to get out of it, or what are my colleagues going to get out of it? If they don't see valuable lessons then people don't report.

Doctor.

The second and more profound concern related to doctors' concerns about managers surveillance and control of their practice. Many doctors suggested reporting had a much more insidious function to monitor medical performance through gathering information about patient harm and, in turn, substandard clinical performance. This view was further supported by the belief, as described above, that managers do not have the knowledge or experience to foster learning, and as such the purpose of incident reporting must be more judgemental and concerned with surveillance. For example, one doctor alluded to Orwell's *1984*, describing reporting as a 'big brother thing'. Other doctors also recognized the way in which the system could further exacerbate tensions between doctors and managers:

There is the potential problem of a them and us situation. People are working hard in the clinical situation. Meanwhile some manager is sitting is an office somewhere looking at the incident form and is likely to come down on us in a judgemental way.

Doctor.

I see it more and more as hemming in and putting the clinician under scrutiny.

Doctor.

Such views touch directly on the micro-political tensions between doctors and managers, especially doctors' anxieties of working in a rationalized and managerial health care system. Reflecting these wider concerns, doctors frequently argued that current changes in the management of patient safety were a further attempt to rein in and challenge medical practice through the extension of more bureaucratic and management-led procedures. These underlying apprehensions might therefore provide a significant, if not insurmountable, obstacle to culture change and increased reporting. They speak directly to the underlying and long-standing conflict between doctors and managers about the relative balance of power and who should be leading services. Resistance to reporting is not only, therefore, a product of blame but an underlying anxiety about the authority of managers to use reports to survey and assess medical performance.

Co-option

Incident reporting and organizational learning therefore faces a conundrum. On the one hand, doctors recognize the value of reporting and will report under certain circumstances. However, on the other hand, they are mindful of the way reporting might be a bureaucratic exercise that extends management authority over their practice. The question that arises therefore is how can these positions be reconciled for the advancement of patient safety? For a number of medical specialties and groups this was achieved by assuming or co-opting responsibility for the new learning systems. In essence, doctors sought to maintain the ideals of clinical freedom, and thereby deal with their anxieties about management, through incorporating new reporting systems within existing collegial systems of performance review. For some doctors, we therefore found a more nuanced relationship with incident reporting, where incident reporting was seen as a useful tool for improving communication and learning, but rather than being coordinated by hospital managers it should be developed locally by medical staff at the front line of care, to the exclusion of managers. Such support for medical leadership around patient safety reflected not only the desire to contribute to more clinically informed decisions around safety, but also to ensure medical authority over these processes and, importantly, to limit managerial encroachment into areas of medical practice.

We found that all doctors involved in the study were accustomed to participating in a range of peer-based forms of performance review, such as clinical audit, ward rounds and morbidity and mortality committees (Freidson 1970, Rosenthal 1995). These were seen as important for improving practice because they involved doctors of similar experience and expertise, and were focused on tangible, local change. Moreover, they were located at the departmental or occupational level, based upon professional membership and therefore safeguarded notions of clinical freedom and autonomy. These activities therefore contrasted starkly with new patient safety systems that were seen as managerial and involving external scrutiny of medical performance. We also found, however, that a number of medical specialties, despite being committed to collegial forms of peer review, had also come to question and have doubts about whether these activities sufficiently engender learning and improvement at a system level:

> We've had these routines handed down to us from when we were in training. Every SHO [Senior House Officer] has to go through them. I still have to go to them. And in some ways they work ... maybe they could be improved.
>
> Doctor.

> I have asked myself what do I actually get from our morbidity and mortality meetings, but then I suppose every once in a while I do learn something new. We

need to be thinking of ways that utilize that information so it's not just a way for us to pull up the ones who make the odd cock-up.

Doctor.

Given the apparent support for, but also quiet questioning of these established practices, we were interested to find that a number of medical specialties had previous experience of using additional forms of quality and risk management, which shared many features with new patient safety reporting systems. For some, these were implemented long before current trends in patient safety and illustrated a long-standing commitment to incremental change and service improvement. Through our research we found that medical specialties such as obstetrics and anaesthesia had, over the previous two decades, established uni-professional, in-house forms of critical incident reporting alongside their established forms of peer review to support local service development and training. The overwhelming view of these systems was that they enhanced but also maintained existing practices around quality improvement and professional regulation:

> We have been reporting for years. I think certainly when you look at the latest report our maternal care seems to have improved, reporting has enabled us to make these targeted improvements.

Doctor.

> Anaesthesia has independently done this for many years before the [hospital]; we have done it for years and years.

Doctor.

We were interested to note that for these doctors, reports were made to a designated department, rather than a hospital-wide risk coordinator, who was therefore seen as working within the local department and therefore was seen as being aligned with doctors rather than management. With the introduction of the new patient safety systems, these doctors took the view that their established systems of incident reporting were largely superior and better suited to medical work. Their response was therefore to decline participation in the new hospital systems, but to share elements of their own data with hospital managers. Significantly, this included data that concealed individual clinicians' details, but was high in clinical content and detail, thereby making it difficult for managers to utilize.

For other medical specialties we also found examples of reporting that exist outside the new systems introduced through the NRLS. These reporting systems involved replicating, or rather adapting, the reporting systems introduced by hospital managers so that they better reflected the current working practices and expectations of doctors. In particular, these were seen as more appropriate for medical work, requiring less time to complete and being more relevant to medical practice.

For these doctors, the development of different reports system or the modification of hospital-wide reporting systems was based upon an ethos of supportive learning and professionalism. There was widespread support for these alternative approaches because clinicians knew all reported information would be kept confidential and not shared with managers. This illustrates the importance of collegiality within medical work, or the idea that doctors of similar experiences and grade, who share similar values and norms, should work together to remedy any problems within their work (Rosenthal 1995, Waring 2005). However, it again raises further questions about the extent to which learning occurs across professional boundaries within more inclusive communities.

Doctors have been found, and perhaps should be encouraged, to embrace new reporting systems through adapting them or assuming responsibility for them within and alongside existing forms of performance review. On the one hand this ensures that patient safety activities align with the ideals of clinical autonomy and limits managerial surveillance of performance. On the other hand it also engenders some form of cultural change towards reporting and provides a model of learning that could be developed and led locally according it greater relevance to clinical staff. The willingness of doctors to embrace elements of the patient safety movement and develop similar practice within and alongside their existing forms of quality control and regulation, further questions the appropriateness of top-down forms of learning. It suggests that models of learning may be more fruitful and have greater medical participation and support when they are initiated and situated within medical practice.

Despite the real potential for fostering learning from below or from within, a number of outstanding questions arise from these findings. Namely, learning typically occurs at the intra-professional and specialty level. That is, doctors working within a given department or area tend to share information with like-minded and professionally commensurate colleagues. Illustrating the homophilly principle, this reinforces tribal or silo-like behaviour and inhibits learning across occupational or organizational boundaries. Given that modern health care relies upon a diverse range of occupational groups working in and contributing to complex care pathways, in particular teamwork settings, the benefits of learning within single occupational silos has limited gains for all those other occupations equally involved in the organization and delivery of care. Furthermore, given that new lines of thinking about human error emphasize the importance of teamwork and interaction with colleagues, this closed-shop approach has limited scope for fostering more widespread inter-professional learning opportunities. In sum, whilst it presents doctors with a new form of learning, it also reinforces professional boundaries and marginalizes other groups from learning activities.

Discussion

Our study suggests the implementation of learning systems, like those developed in aviation or petrochemicals, is not a straight forward activity with automatically positive outcomes for service improvement. Rather it is a highly contested and political process that talks to the underlying tensions between professionals and managers. As we show, the idea of establishing procedures that better capture information about the threats to patient safety so that they can be used to inform organizational change remains problematic. For those working within the health care sector, especially doctors, the implementation of centralized managerial systems is seen as an anathema or affront to the cultural ideals and expectations around learning, professional development, the disclosure of information and notions of collegiality. This produces a range of reactions from doctors, from forms of participation at the margins, to more significant expressions of resistance and, more significantly, examples of co-option.

To help us better understand these reactions we can look to ideas and debates within the field of organizational learning (Easterby-Smith and Lyles 2005). Structured forms of learning associated with what is called Knowledge Management (KM) have come to strongly influence management thinking and now health policy (Reason 2000). These have grown in popularity, in part because of their contributions to safety in other industries, but also because of their growing application through information technologies. As outlined above, these promise organizations with a systematic way of marshalling knowledge through three common stages of knowledge accumulation, knowledge storage and analysis and knowledge leverage. As a method of organizational learning, KM can be regarded as an overtly managerial and technocratic approach (Currie et al. 2008). Elaborating this, it is often developed, implemented and led by managers, within layers of upward accountability, and tied to performance objectives that are largely managerial in nature. Despite seeking to foster learning and improved ways of working, the managerial nature of KM can mean that it fails to truly acknowledge or come to terms with the more socio-cultural and political realities of knowledge and learning within organizations.

Other perspectives on organizational learning help us to better understand the socio-cultural and political world revealed above. Where KM is associated with the practical management of knowledge as a technical solution or fix, this alternate perspective offers a more critical understanding of learning within complex organizational and occupational settings. In particular, it shows how knowledge sharing and learning are complex social activities that cannot easily be managed or controlled. Studies show how knowledge itself is often situated within occupational practice, being tacit, and embedded within social interaction (Lave and Wenger 1991). This can mean that it is often difficult to capture, codify or share this knowledge through centralized systems that are premised on explicit and often tangible or abstract facts or events. Developing the idea that knowledge and learning are situated, research also reveals the important role played by occupational cultures in shaping and reinforcing not only knowledge, but also social practice. That is, occupational groups are often characterized by strong and deeply embedded values and norms that can reinforce normal, customary or socialized ways of working. This suggests therefore, that one occupational group may vary from another occupational group with regards to what information is valued as important and worthy of communication, together with the normal and anticipated ways of conveying and reacting to this information. This implies that learning within organizations is often more fruitful when it is situated within everyday social practices rather than centralized through managerial processes (Lave and Wenger 1991). As noted above, however, caution should be taken if supporting these bottom-up approaches to ensure that they are inclusive of all relevant professional groups and not reinforcing tribal-like behaviours and maintaining jurisdictional boundaries.

A related line of analysis relates to the sociopolitical dimension of learning. From this perspective, knowledge is seen as a powerful resource that not only informs the technical aspects of work practice, but contributes to the formation and maintenance of jurisdictional boundaries, claims to expertise and occupational identities (Freidson 1970). There are well established sociological literatures, both within the areas of the professions and medical sociology, that illustrate how the processes of professional socialization are closely associated with the acquisition of both explicit and tacit knowledge related to the technical and non-technical dimensions of work (Freidson 1970). Furthermore, control of this knowledge provides a basis for securing occupational jurisdiction in the competitive social division of labour; providing occupational groups within exclusive domains of practice and increased levels of status (Abbott 1988). Notwithstanding a range of social, legal and organizational factors that help to create and reinforce this role, professional discretion or autonomy is largely premised on the acquisition, control and effective utilization of expert or indeterminate knowledge, as those without this knowledge are limited in the extent to which they can direct or evaluate legitimately the application of this knowledge in professional practice (Abbott 1988).

The complex relationship between professional knowledge and practice is exemplified by the legitimacy and power of the medical profession. The inherent asymmetries of knowledge around health and illness can been seen in the professions enduring claims to clinical freedom or autonomy, as well as the status differential within the doctor–patient relationship. Although it remains important to acknowledge that there are clear variations between health care professions, with significant differences witnessed between medical and other occupational groups, the ability of some professions, such as medicine, to more effectively guard areas of its knowledge from outside groups has been richly described in sociological research, where collegial groupings provide the primary focus for socialization, learning and the setting of professional expectations (Rosenthal 1995). With specific relevance to issues of patient safety, it is within these collegial groupings or communities of practice that issues of clinical risk are raised, shared and controlled so as to reinforce professional status. Such silo-type communities have increasingly come to the fore of patient safety policies, particularly following the series of major scandals of patient harm and clinical error, and it is perhaps these silos that policies are really attempting to overcome.

Given the important role played by knowledge in the maintenance of occupational status and legitimacy, efforts to manage knowledge in the pursuit of organizational learning can be interpreted as a major challenge to the foundations of occupational status and legitimacy. This is because it enables organizational leaders to acquire, store and utilize knowledge that has been central to the formation of occupational roles and jurisdictional boundaries. Elaborating this line of thinking, the organizational learning perspective highlights how knowledge management systems can constitute a managerial strategy for wresting the control and application of knowledge towards organizational, as opposed to occupational priorities (Wilmott 2000). KM reflects the long-standing conflict between capital and labour as the former seeks out new ways of ordering the latter. In other words, KM provides management with techniques for acquiring and utilizing knowledge that has been traditionally associated with the expert aspects of work and beyond the scope of direct management intervention. By externalizing the control of knowledge in this way managers have the opportunity for challenging established occupational boundaries and areas of exclusivity, in particular, making it more feasible to supervise and direct work activities.

This political dimension of learning is particularly relevant in the case of the UK patient safety reforms. It becomes immediately apparent that the NRLS represents a mechanism to lever clinical knowledge towards, although not exclusively, managerial priorities. Moreover, this political dimension becomes even more pronounced when the NRLS is located within wider debates about the management and regulation of medical practice and autonomy. Over the last 30 years much has been written about the growth of managerial roles and responsibilities within the organization and delivery of health care (Harrison and McDonald 2008). The rationalizing tendencies of these corporate groups towards cost-savings and the more efficient organization of clinical services have been interpreted as introducing countervailing powers within health care that cut a swathe across established lines of medical power and influence. As suggested above, it is this tension between doctors and managers that beguiles the implementation of learning systems within health care, but also encourages doctors to rethink and develop their existing systems of learning within their existing occupational boundaries. Reflecting the idea that learning is a social activity (Lave and Wenger 1991), we find some degree of encouragement from those doctors that attempt to implement more robust forms of learning within or alongside their collegial practice. This demonstrates not only the willingness of some doctors to respond positively to the wider patient safety agenda, but also to question and change their existing systems. Learning at the local or departmental level perhaps delivers change that is more attuned to the needs of professionals whilst reinforcing the occupational control of knowledge and limiting managerial encroachment. Whilst such efforts should clearly be supported, questions remain about the degree to which these activities facilitate change across occupational boundaries and at a wider organizational level. Without the sharing of knowledge more widely doubts emerge about the extent to which lessons can be shared between professional groups, health care providers or at a service-wide level.

The answer, therefore, may be to find ways in which to locate new models of learning within the day-to-day culture and world of professional practice, so that control and ownership remains local. However, this is not an argument for returning power or authority back to a single occupational groups, such as medicine, but rather for fostering more robust forms of learning across and between those occupations involved in the day-to-day world of care provision; those who make the difficult clinical decisions and care for patients; those who often know more about clinical risk and know best how to make safety improvements. As shown by the example of doctors, new opportunities for learning can be actively taken up and adapted at the local level, but worryingly there is a need to challenge the growth of uni-professional models, as shown in this chapter, and instead establish more team-based approaches that are inclusive of all relevant groups. This is important to counter learning that simply reinforces the power and status of one group at the expense of others. Such systems must also offer opportunities for sharing lessons upwards and outwards, in a way that is driven by professionals and supported by managers. So the lessons developed within one service area or team can be disseminated more widely. Only then are strong professional groups who privilege and guard knowledge about their clinical practice likely to favour sharing this knowledge with others.

References

Abbott, A. 1988. *The System of Professions*. Chicago: University of Chicago Press.

Currie, G., Waring, J. and Finn, R. 2008. The limits of knowledge management for public sector modernisation. The case of patient safety and quality. *Public Administration*, 86(2), 363–385.

Department of Health. 2000. *An Organization with a Memory*. London: TSO.

Easterby-Smith, M. and Lyles, M. 2005. Introduction: watersheds of organizational learning and knowledge management. In: Easterby-Smith, M. and Lyles, M. (eds) *The Blackwell Handbook of Organizational Learning and Knowledge Management*. Oxford: Blackwell, pp. 1–17.

Flynn, R. 2004. Soft-bureaucracy, governmentality and clinical governance: theoretical approaches to emergent policy. In: Gray, A. and Harrison, S. (eds) *Governing Medicine*. Maidenhead: Open University Press, pp. 11–26.

Freidson, E. 1970. *The Profession of Medicine*. New York: Harper Row.

Harrison, S. 2004. Governing medicine: governance, science and practice. In: Gray, A. and Harrison, S. (eds) *Governing Medicine*. Maidenhead: Open University Press, pp. 180–187.

Harrison, S. and McDonald, R. 2008. *The Politics of Healthcare in Britain.* London: Sage.

Institute of Medicine. 1999. *To Err is Human.* Washington: IoM.

Kennedy, I. 2001. *The Bristol Royal Infirmary Inquiry.* London: TSO.

Lave, J. and Wenger, E. 1991. *Situated Learning: Legitimate Peripheral Participation.* Cambridge: Cambridge University Press.

Lawrence, T., Mauws, M., Dyck, B. and Kleyson, R. 2005. The politics of organizational learning: integrating power into the 4I framework. *Academy of Management Review*, 301(1), 180–191.

Light, D. 1995. Countervailing powers: a framework for professions in transition. In: Johnson, T., Larkin, G. and Saks, M. (eds) *Health Professions and the State in Europe.* London: Routledge, pp. 25–43.

National Patient Safety Agency. 2003. *Seven Steps to Patient Safety.* London: NPSA.

Reason, J. 1997. *Managing the Risks of Organizational Accidents.* Aldershot: Ashgate.

Reason, J. (2000) Human error: models and management. *British Medical Journal*, 320, 768–770.

Reason, J. and Hobbs, A. 2003. *Managing Maintenance Error: A Practice Guide.* Aldershot: Ashgate.

Rosenthal, M. 1995. *The Incompetent Doctor.* Maidenhead: Open University Press.

Smith, J. 2004. *The Shipman Inquiry, Vol. 4.* London: TSO.

Walshe, K. 1999. Medical accidents in the UK: a wasted opportunity for improvement. In: Rosenthal, M., Mulcahy, L. and Lloyd-Bostock, S. (eds) *Medical Mishaps.* Maidenhead: Open University Press, pp. 59–73.

Waring, J. 2005. Beyond blame: cultural barriers to medical reporting. *Social Science and Medicine*, 60, 1927–1935.

Willis, P. 1977. *Learning to Labour.* New York: Columbia University Press.

Willmott, H. 2000. From knowledge to learning. In: Hull, R., Chumer, M. and Willmott, H. (eds), *Managing Knowledge: Critical Investigations of Work and Learning.* Basingstoke: MacMillan, pp. 216–231.

World Health Organisation. 2004. *World Alliance for Patient Safety.* Geneva: WHO.

Chapter 8

Exploring the Contributions of Professional-Practice Networks to Knowledge Sharing, Problem-Solving and Patient Safety

Simon Bishop and Justin Waring

It is widely accepted that improvements in patient safety are often found in enhanced communication amongst health care professionals. Clinicians need to learn about the threats to patient safety through openly sharing knowledge about these events so as to bring about both necessary change in practice and more widespread organizational learning. Attempts to embed knowledge sharing and learning within health care can be seen, for example, with the development and adoption of formal reporting and knowledge management systems (see National Patient Safety Agency 2003). These have drawn upon experiences in other hazardous industries where they have been developed to dramatically reduce the incidence of adverse events (Weick and Sutcliffe 2001). While these have contributed to patient safety in certain instances, their contribution to more widespread learning is unclear, as demonstrated by variable levels of reporting. One possible reason for the low levels of success is the endurance of alternative communities or networks of communication that are shaped less by managerially designed systems of information distribution and more by the activities of clinical practice and professional allegiance (Braithwaite et al. 2009). These informal networks are usually formed organically over time without explicit direction or management. Although they might be seen as a hindrance to learning because they serve to hoard or conceal knowledge within professional silos or clinical 'cliques' (Kennedy 2001), there is widespread agreement that such networks or communities of practices provide a significant basis for learning (Lave and Wenger 1991).

A small number of studies consider the patterns, formation and outcomes of different types of communities or 'natural networks' in health care (Scott et al. 2005, Tagliaventi and Mattarelli 2006, Creswick et al. 2010). These identify some important features of clinical networks, such as the way joint practice helps build strong interpersonal ties and how professional groupings shape interaction. However, the contribution of such natural networks to the production of quality and safety in health care is under-researched. Braithwaite et al. (2009) identify this as a key gap in our current understanding of quality improvement. They argue that service transformation and improvement relies upon a complex system of well-established clinical communities and teams, and that clinicians work best when they are allowed to work in groupings of their own choosing and interest. An important task for those interested in quality improvement is to uncover the properties of these networks, including the patterns of interaction, the basis of formation and the common values, and to understand how these can be harnessed to share safe practices in ways that appeal intrinsically to those involved in delivering care. Accordingly, it might be suggested that these natural or organic networks are often better suited to the sharing of knowledge amongst clinicians than more managed or mechanistic systems of reporting.

In this chapter we seek to deepen our understanding and appreciation of how these professional-practice networks might contribute to patient safety, especially through providing an informal, rapid and service-facing basis for problem-solving and decision-making. The chapter reports on the findings of a mixed-method study of communication and patient safety. The study combines social network analysis (SNA) to determine the patterns of interactions amongst clinicians, specifically in relation to problem-solving and the safe completion of work, together with ethnographic observations of work processes and cultures. One common view of SNA is that is better suited to identifying the relationships (ties) between actors (nodes) but not at explaining how they form, function or contribute to practice (Scott 2000). As such, observations over a period of 18 months help to compliment this data. This type of study is important because, although communication activities have been found to take the majority of clinicians' time in acute care settings (Coiera et al. 2002), the content and contribution of communication is currently poorly understood. The chapter begins by outlining and questioning the current approaches to improving patient safety associated with top-down managerial initiatives. It goes on to elaborate the salient features and potential benefits of naturally occurring social networks, before showing from our findings how such professional-practice networks are integral to problem-solving and safe working. The discussion and conclusion focuses on how the results might promote certain practices, with reference to theoretical work on communities of practice (Lave and Wenger 1991).

The Limits of Formal Learning Systems

There is a consensus that patient safety can be improved through higher standards of communication. Equally, there is considerable evidence that a lack of information sharing, professional secrecy and a failure to learn from mistakes are partially to blame for serious incidents and routine patient safety failings (Helmreich 2000, Neale et al. 2001). Communication and knowledge sharing are therefore central factors in determining the quality of care processes and outcomes.

Current approaches to improving communication around patient safety are largely shaped by two popular managerial concepts. First is the notion of the 'learning organization' (Senge 1996). This refers to the idea of an organization that habitually captures, codifies, disseminates and puts into practice lessons learned on the 'front line'. In this view, the degree to which an organization adapts and changes in response to new information is central to its success. This is seen as essential because it promises to remove the common blocks to learning in health care, gaining the collective input of all workers, building open cultures and new relationships (Birleson 1998). Second is the idea of the 'high reliability system'. This refers to those, often high-risk organizations that have been found to improve their safety record through actively identifying and controlling procedural and operational risks through organizational design, heightened awareness, operational protocols and continually updating procedures in response to failures or warnings (Weick and Sutcliffe 2001).

The influence of these ideas can be seen in current global approaches to patient safety. Policy makers have attempted to purposefully design and promote more formal communication systems explicitly aimed at fostering organization learning. For instance, new information technologies, checking procedures, reporting systems and standardized categorizations of errors have been developed and widely adopted to support communication, improved clinical safety and organizational learning (Chang et al. 2005). Wilson et al. (2005) promote several team-level communication behaviours to improve safety, including 'closed loop' communication checks in which both the sending and receipt of information is formally recorded; peer monitoring of performance with feedback of observations; and allowing junior team members to voice concerns where their expertise warrants. Similarly, Firth-Cozens (2001) describes the managerial approaches to improve safety culture, for example through changing reward structures, building patient safety questions into decision-making and leadership activities associated with a safety culture.

Although there is evidence that reporting interventions has led to the reduction of adverse outcomes in some instances (Kaushal et al. 2003), there remains limited evidence for the successful translation of safety practices developed outside of health care (AHRQ 2001). There is evidence, for example, that incident reporting systems, the primary approach for sharing safety knowledge and fostering organizational learning, have variable staff participation (Lawton and Parker 2002, Waring 2005, Waring and Currie Chapter 7 this volume). In short, such systems only capture a fracture of the safety knowledge that permeates and circulates the clinical workplace. In addition, the adoption of formal management systems intended to shape knowledge practices does not automatically lead to health professionals changing their real-life activities (Finn et al. 2010). One potential reason for the growing evidence is the existence of pre-existing networks of communication, namely the patterns of interpersonal interaction between health care professionals through which information is routinely, often implicitly shared throughout the working day. Attempts to introduce more formalized, standardized and managerial systems of knowledge sharing might be seen as overlapping with or even conflicting with the more informal, collegial and practice-based networks of communication that feature in everyday clinical work.

Professional-practice Networks

Recognizing the potential limits of formal reporting systems, Braithwaite et al. (2009) highlight the possibilities of natural networks for patient safety. They argue that while mandated communication systems may be useful for certain tasks, such as logistical and infrastructure management, there is a tendency to forget the organic or natural networks between health professionals that routinely ensure the safety of day-to-day care delivery. Health care services are produced by 'webs of humans connected personally or via technologies, interacting in multiple ways' (Braithwaite et al. 2009: 37). Unlike formal reporting systems, these communities of practice evolve over time without formal direction or control, they operate on the basis of mutual and voluntary participation, have high levels of trust, involve a tacit shared understanding of work tasks and the norms of interaction and can be called upon in response to the multifarious challenges of care delivery. Braithwaite et al. also highlight the intrinsic appeal of these networks to their members, where the network properties naturally develop from the discretion of individual members interacting over time. This chimes with much of the research on knowledge sharing networks, where interpersonal judgements of, for example, trustworthiness, shared interest and expertise are found to shape knowledge sharing about formal organizational roles (Borgatti and Cross 2003).

The existence of informal social networks is often mentioned in literature on safety, but is equally regarded as an idiosyncrasy of the health sector, or alternatively as actively preventing improvements in safety. Firth-Cozen (2001) notes the role alliances play in sharing information, for example influencing who is blamed for mistakes. Similarly, Rosenthal (1995) highlights how small groups of like-minded doctors work to manage clinical risks behind closed doors. In general, such communities are associated with secrecy, unaccountability and bad practice, and therefore perceived as running counter to the goal of patient safety. For example, spreading information only within a particular professional group is commonly seen as knowledge hoarding and serving self-interest rather than promoting learning (Bontis and Sorenko 2009). In addition, studies have illustrated how networks with high-trust relationships may counteract efforts to purposefully shape the collection and distribution of information amongst health care services (Currie and Suhomlinova 2006). As such, considerable attention has been paid to the negative or dark side of these alliances or 'cliques' and their need to be managed in the pursuit of patient safety.

In light of this view, there has been limited empirical study of how informal networks of front line staff contribute to patient safety. What is needed, according to Braithwaite et al., is a fuller recognition of the role played by natural networks in the production of health care. They argue that 'a bottom-up strategy led by clinicians is badly needed to balance the predominantly top-down approaches which frequently result in only modest improvements which are difficult to sustain' (Braithwaite et al. 2009: 37).

This might involve, for instance, returning to the wider literature on social networks which has been long-established in the anthropological and sociology study of communities (Scott 2000). Such research considers the reasons why certain patterns of interpersonal relationships emerge, the characteristics and features of such relationships and how different patterns result in different social capacities such as providing support or spreading information (Scott 2000). Importantly, studies of enduring community networks illustrate how the patterns of everyday interaction strongly alter the attitudes and beliefs of individual actors (Rice and Aydin 1991), their preferences and tastes (Lewis et al. 2008), their current choices of activities (Warde et al. 2005), as well as their life opportunities and future prospects (Granovetter 1973, Putnam 1995). Studies of social networks have also found that strong, enduring interpersonal relationships are most commonly formed between those with demographic similarities or kinship (Lazarsfeld and Merton 1954), linguistic compatibility (March and Simon 1958), shared commercial interests (Blok 1973), or common historical circumstances (Menjivar 1995).

With reference to knowledge sharing and organizational learning, research also shows how network characteristics can affect the flow of information. Most frequently these highlight the importance of trust (Lorenz 1989, Levin and Cross 2004), as well as factors such as the frequency of interaction and a shared worldview. Similarly, the overall pattern of relationships within a group has been found to shape knowledge sharing. Important concepts here include the overall 'density' of relationships within a group, how centrally the network converges around high-status members, and the relationship between 'core' and 'periphery' members (Wasserman and Faust 1994, Scott 2000). These play an important role in how quickly information is likely to spread within and around a social community. For example, research identifies key people occupying certain network positions, such as 'boundary spanners' or 'knowledge brokers' (Williams 2002) that link otherwise unconnected groups.

Only a small number of studies have begun to map the real-life networks of interaction within health care (Cott 1997, West et al. 1999, Scott et al. 2005). For example, Tagliaventi and Mattarelli's (2006) study of communication networks within a radiation oncology unit identified frequent interactions between number of different professions, including surgeons, physicians, nurses and technicians. In line with previous understanding, knowledge sharing was most common and intense within professional groups, for example, nurse to nurse, but it was also found that interprofessional sharing did occur under certain conditions. Namely, when people from different professional groups work side-by-side in everyday operational tasks, and when they share common values about the organizational unit, or 'ideological consensus' (Hudson 2004). Similarly, Creswick et al.'s (2010) study within an emergency department highlighted the central role played by junior doctors and nursing staff in helping medical colleagues solve work-related problems. Looking further at the differences between occupational groups, West et al. (1999) looked at the dense network of Directors of Medicine versus the more dispersed networks of Directors of Nursing, concluding that these lead to different capacities for disseminating information and inducing change amongst the workforce.

Building on these studies, our research investigated the contribution of professional-practice networks to patient safety through exploring how information is understood and shared within these communities, and how subsequent safety-related activities are carried out. Interpersonal networks may affect safe practice in many ways. For example, increased levels of trust may lead clinicians to share important or sensitive information or seek out advice and guidance. Rather than knowledge hoarding and professional elitism, there is a possibility that such relationships are important filters to help deal with high volumes of information and might therefore facilitate timely decision-making close to the front line. Finally, these professional-practice networks may well overlap with formal reporting or learning systems and lead to certain events being recorded more accurately. Understanding these networks is therefore an important part of understanding the day-to-day features of health care work and our work in this area answers Braithwaite and colleagues' (2009) call for greater study of naturally occurring professional-practice networks in health and their contribution to the production of safe health care.

The Study

Our study focused on knowledge sharing within the professional-practice networks of two day-surgery units (DSUs) in the English NHS. Given known sensitivities around patient safety, the study took as its primary focus the sharing of knowledge involved in day-to-day 'problem-solving'. Pilot research suggested that questions related to directly to communication about patient safety events were poorly interpreted by participants and response rates were negatively affected by concerns about fear of blame, for example participants thought they should mention only formal reporting channels. Moreover, a sole focus on patient safety events tended to focus on reactive communications, such as reporting, rather than more proactive forms of knowledge sharing that are involved in the maintenance of safe working conditions. As such, the study investigated patterns of knowledge sharing involved in day-to-day problem-solving. This involved a survey that asked respondents to name the departmental colleagues whom they commonly sought knowledge from when solving a problem that interfered with the successful and safe completion of work.

The study approach was a mix of statistical and ethnographic social network analysis (SNA). SNA examines the patterns of relationships or 'ties' between people, groups and organizations (Scott 2000, Granovetter 1973). It has a wide variety of applications, such as exploring kinship or employment networks, and can involve a range of methods, from surveys to analysis of historical documents. In practice, SNA usually has a particular empirical focus to help nuance and specify the type of relationships being studied given that social groups occupy a variety of different, overlapping and sometimes competing social networks, for example family and work networks. For our study we focused on how and with whom knowledge was shared in the context of problem-solving, in other words, who do members of a workplace community seek out when trying to solve a problem? A standard SNA survey was administered to all members of both DSUs (DSU#1 n = 59, 80 per cent response rate; DSU#2 n = 47, 85 per cent response rate), asking participants to list those individuals they commonly shared information with when seeking to solve a problem that interfered with the successful and safe completion of work. In order to distinguish between the 'strength' of these relationships, respondents rated on a five-point Likert scale each named person on relational characteristics found in previous SNA studies to affect the extent of knowledge sharing (Borgatti and Cross 2003). This includes measures for frequency, availability, responsiveness, approachability and trust, which together provided valued network data on the problem-solving network.

To better understand how, when and in what context knowledge was shared during problem-solving, qualitative observations and interviews were also carried out with clinicians in both DSUs. This involved semi-structured face-to-face interviews (64) and observations of day-to-day working practices over 18 months. Interviews included five vignettes asking participants to identify 'who', 'when', 'how' and 'why' they would share knowledge in situations such as delays, missing information, patient harm and resource shortages. These situations were based on recognized risk factors in surgery (Catchpole et al. 2007, Waring et al. 2007), worded in consultation with an advisory panel of health care professionals. This qualitative stage was used to explore the survey findings in greater depth, such as what types of knowledge were exchanged and when.

Results

In both DSUs, the problem-solving networks were large and complex. Although there were clear differences in the shape and character of the communication networks between the two sites, there were also a number of interesting similarities and common themes. Drawing together results from the surveys and qualitative study, our findings show both important benefits and drawbacks to informal knowledge networks as a means of sharing knowledge on patient safety.

The SNA survey data revealed that more frequent and stronger levels of communication were linked to a number of widely recognized factors (Borgatti and Cross 2003). These include the frequency of contact between individuals, higher levels of trust, homophily of professional group, better understanding of others' expertise and long tenure were all positively related to the occurrence of knowledge sharing between any two individuals. Further, the formal roles people held, such as team leader or clinical manager, and their hierarchical status also appeared to affect the degree to which people sought them out for information and advice. For example, the nursing grade was positively correlated with centrality in the network. This would suggest that higher-ranking nurses played a more important role in knowledge sharing.

Particularly important, and in line with findings from previous studies, we found that knowledge tended to be shared more freely amongst individuals within rather than between professional group. Although there are many caveats to this – discussed below – professional membership played a key role in shaping who clinicians shared knowledge within the context of problem-solving. The divide or gap between groups was most evident in the network position of surgeons and anaesthetists. Despite the fact that these professionals are integral to the organization and delivery of surgical care, it was evident that knowledge sharing between surgical and anaesthetic staff, both amongst themselves and with other clinicians, was uniformly less than for the other groups. This homophily of knowledge sharing raises potential challenges for problem-solving. If problems are most freely discussed within groups, information may not so readily flow to group outsiders and interprofessional problems might not be addressed.

As well as professional divisions, there was also a gap between 'core' and 'periphery' DSU staff. In general, higher levels of knowledge sharing were reported between those who worked together more frequently, for example on a day-to-day basis. For example, knowledge sharing *between* nurses, operating department practitioners (ODPs) and health care assistants (HCAs) was almost as common as knowledge sharing *within* these professional groups. During observations, these 'core', often non-medical staff, engaged in constant communication throughout the working day as they worked side-by-side making decisions, preparing patients and equipment and delivering surgical care. These staff remained in continual dialogue across various clinical settings: at the ward desk, in the pre-assessment rooms, during theatre changeovers, where they often discussed issues relating to safety and quality, including immediate patient care, staffing and equipment, specific events and the general quality of the service. It was evident that these exchanges were underpinned by a sense of camaraderie and collegiality amongst the core staff, for example rising in intensity during busy periods as staff jointly recognized the need to 'get things done quickly'. These non-medical groups tended to view themselves as being constitutive of the DSU staff, distinct from the managers or the doctors. Respondents from these occupational groups referred to themselves as 'us' or 'the staff' and reported generally high levels of trust, shared understanding and capacity for problem-solving.

The close day-to-day contact between these individuals allowed the staff to recognize and understand each others' skills and abilities, as well as reinforce shared goals, values and norms about work and working relationships. Across the respondents, this intimate knowledge of colleagues working practices was seen as vitally important for working on joint tasks, helping them judge task timings, capabilities and who to seek out in relation to particular problems. This suggests that frequency of contact can contribute to strong knowledge sharing ties, overcoming potential professional barriers. Moreover, this collaborative practice enabled staff to develop shared knowledge and language about their work, to understand how others worked, how they could contribute to problem-solving and to foster levels of trust between clinicians. It was widely felt that an intricate knowledge of colleagues practice was beneficial to effective working and problem-solving. As a qualification to this, even amongst these groups, perceived distinctions could occasionally be seen to surface. For example, issues of training and expertise were cited as reasons why certain issues were kept within-group. Higher-status groups such as theatre nurses cited their specialist expertise as a reason why certain issues were best dealt with amongst professional peers:

> I have seen status issues and they are largely because due to our qualifications there are certain actions that we can or can't take. A classic one would be that an ODP can't do certain things that I can do as a nurse.

Theatre Nurse 5.

In contrast with the close connections amongst the 'core' staff, surgical, anaesthetic and many administrative staff tended to be on the periphery of the network. Unlike the nurses and ODPs, surgeons and anaesthetists were seen as only 'visiting' the DSU once or twice a week to undertake their allocated theatre work. This transitory work within the DSUs meant that these individuals were less embedded within the networks of knowledge sharing and had not built upon the strong ties as widely found amongst the core staff. As such, there was usually less opportunity for informal communication between medics and non-medical staff, with surgeons tending not to use the communal areas and staff lounge. In turn, it was found that these clinicians tended to rely upon more specific individual contacts or relationships to distribute and acquire information in the context of problem-solving, for example interacting with the service managers or lead nurses without automatically engaging the wider staff group. Equally, nurses and ODPs were less willing to engage these 'visitors' in non-goal-orientated conversation or confront them directly with a problem:

> What makes it impossible is the personality of the surgeon because we do have some people who are most obnoxious and the minute they get obnoxious I won't take it and I just go and get the manager in.

Theatre Nurse 2.

While these patterns of knowledge sharing might reflect established hierarchies between health care professionals, our study indicated this was reinforced by the established working patterns and necessities of practice in the DSU. Although it is difficult to separate cause and effect, there was some reason to suggest that the working patterns and the lack of opportunity to build strong interpersonal relationships exacerbated the barriers to interprofessional knowledge sharing. For example, new medics and infrequent visitors were seen to have little knowledge of the layout of the department or who to ask for basic information about the day's planned activities.

Mitigating the divide between occupational groups was the role of managers and senior nurses who acted as key hubs, coordinators or knowledge brokers with each DSU. Survey results showed how the most senior nurse managers were the most central people in the networks. Within the DSUs the senior nurses could be seen as the 'natural hubs [who] disproportionately influence policies events and practices' (Braithwaite et al., 2009: 38). Qualitative data suggested how their role and practice gave them the legitimacy to bridge different groups. In both DSUs, the senior nurses had worked in their respective units for longer than 10 years and were seen as having knowledge 'valued by both sides' (Surgeon 2). On one hand they were seen by medics as important sources of information and knowledgeable about the workings of the department, including interpersonal issues, the skills of staff members, bureaucratic procedures and generally how to get things done. As such, surgeons and anaesthetists regarded these senior nurses as the primary contact points for dealing with problems and ensuring the smooth running of the service. On the other hand, these senior nurses were also seen by nurses and ODPs as being involved and embedded in daily practice and aware of the common stresses and frustrations that could make day-to-day practice problematic. They were therefore almost universally seen as legitimate in representing the views and practices across the department. Responding to a question about dealing with problems in scheduling an anaesthetist stated:

> I might go to the secretary, but if I think there is not enough is being done I will speak to [the senior nurse] and say 'what about this'. She is the ultimate master of what happens and how things are actually being done. She is looking at the waiting lists and all of her staff as well.

> Anaesthetist 1.

While other nursing staff may have hesitated in expressing concerns or discussing problems with medical staff, lead nurses were seen as able to legitimately represent their views:

> I am not a consultant general surgeon and they are, but there are certain times that you consider dangerous and then it is a case of having to be accountable for what you do and I would say that if you are not comfortable or confident to deal with it yourself then it shouldn't be ignored, but I would go and speak to the [lead nurse].

> Theatre Nurse 11.

Based on the features noted above, informal professional-practice networks can be seen as impacting both positively and negatively on problem-solving, and potentially on patient safety. On the one hand, personal contacts were seen by respondents as the most important sources of patient safety information and essential for the delivery of safe care. On the other hand, these networks shape who shares knowledge with whom, suggesting some people or groups are privileged in their access to certain knowledge, whereas other people or groups are likely to be left out.

One consequence of this is that some problems, indeed safety issues, were observed as being resolved quickly in the context of clinical practice, whereas others required purposeful activities to be developed post hoc to search for solutions. To give examples of each, one common problem faced by both DSUs was the appropriate distribution of nursing staff between pre-operative areas, theatres and recovery areas as workload fluctuated during the working day. Although broad parameters and tasks were allocated and managed by managers and nurse leaders, many of these fluctuations were accommodated and controlled by the nursing and ODP staff on the ground. This capacity to deal with uncertainty and change was based on their knowledge of the most appropriate clinicians to seek out for guidance and advice at the required time or stage within the care process. Sharing knowledge about, and ultimately collaborating to control for the potential risks to safe care delivery through informal communications channels meant that safe staffing levels could be maintained efficiently. However, this common problem-solving event could be complicated when surgeons and anaesthetists made additional requirements for staffing arrangement, for example, using specialist equipment, adding or changing patients on the surgical list or extending the length of surgery beyond the usual operating period. In such cases, the delivery of surgical care required theatre staff with particular skills, capabilities or experience that could not easily be identified by surgical or anaesthetic staff given their lack of familiarity with departmental skill-mix. Without knowledge of each nurse, their skills, workloads and working patterns, doctors were therefore unable to approach these individuals informally for help at a given time. To resolve this, a formal request would usually be made to the theatre manager or lead nurse, prior to the start of surgery, to arrange for certain nurse teams to be in place for the duration of specific lists. While this often solved the problem, it also led to reduction in flexibility as nurses tied to particular lists were then unable to rotate around the department, and also caused friction when requests were not fulfilled, for example due to absence or sickness.

In general, the results show how informal professional-practice networks enable knowledge about problems and safety to be mobilized and shared quickly. Informal knowledge sharing was continuous and essential for all aspects of health care practice. However, the drivers of group exchange and knowledge sharing 'within' group, such as intricate awareness of others' skills, high levels of trust and shared language, were also the barriers to 'without' or between group exchange. As has previously been noted, it would be unfeasible for each individual to invest the time and energy to build strong ties with all other network members, across all groups (Burt 1982). Nevertheless, informal knowledge sharing produces problem-solving, learning and safety in ways that formal systems cannot. Specifically, knowledge sharing is close to the action and is integral to resilient safe practice. However, it can also be said that in certain instances more conscious and formal systems may be required to bridge the gaps in informal networks, especially those between groups. These may solve certain problems, but they should not be seen as replacing informal knowledge sharing and may indeed create different issues and challenges of their own.

Discussion

Research and policy in the area of patient safety advocate the importance of both interpersonal communication in improving teamwork and safe care delivery, and also formal systems of knowledge sharing to foster systemic learning and safety improvement. Much of the existing literature portrays clinical communities or cliques as countering communication, learning and safety, given compelling evidence of knowledge hoarding and collusion in the wake of safety events. As such, much attention has been given to the role of checklists and incident reporting procedures to improve knowledge sharing and patient safety. However, there is growing attention to the potential positive, even unsung, contribution that informal patterns or networks of communication make to day-to-day care organization and delivery. As demonstrated in this chapter, knowledge often flows freely and quickly amongst clinicians within informal networks, and these have a significant role in decision-making, problem-solving and patient safety. Building on this relatively small literature, our chapter illustrates that these engrained patterns of knowledge sharing are based upon high degrees of trust, shared understanding of clinical knowledge and roles, common purpose and awareness of operational processes and an underlying sense of collegiality or camaraderie. Clearly, these attributes have both positive and negative implications. As we show, there are clear boundaries between core and peripheral groups that reflect not only occupational boundaries and status hierarchies, but also established patterns of working in the delivery of day surgery. Whilst knowledge is exchanged and mobilized quickly for non-medical or core groups, there are inherent gaps in the flow of knowledge between the core (non-medical) and the periphery (medical) groups. However, our analysis also shows how these gaps are mediated, especially through the work of nurse leaders, managers and medical representatives who can provide individual brokers to bridge and assist the flow of knowledge between staff groups.

Our findings lead us to suggest that efforts to increase safety should not solely focus on checklist, formal reporting and managerially imposed systems. As Vincent et al. (2010) point out, many of the studies of high reliability organizations involve military personal, those socialized to work in strict hierarchy and those that adhere to precise routines. Conversely, health care represents a unique multi-professional environment involving heterogeneous interests, contested relationships between groups and a wide variety of standards and performance objectives even within a single organization. These ambiguities in the nature of health care work may indeed require a greater degree of face-to-face, open-ended discussion to reach acceptable solutions to problems (Coiera and Tombes 1998). Neither explicit organizational charts nor imposed formal reporting systems are likely to tell the whole story of how safety-related activities are enacted and understood. There should therefore be greater focus on acknowledging and supporting informal professional-practice networks in the promotion of patient safety, for example recognizing important peripheral actors and bringing them into more frequent contact with those who informally and tacitly shape the agenda within a particular department. Rather than concentrating on changing individual behaviours or encouraging clinicians to respond to safety events merely through formal channels, there could be a greater emphasis on spreading messages in ways that take advantage of existing real-life social activities. While these may differ between each case, a first step lies in recognizing informal social networks as an essential and inevitable part of working life, rather than solely a hindrance to safe care.

An important contribution of social network study is its ability to direct attention towards the current or potential gaps in care delivery. As Cook et al. (2000) point out, gaps occur in many areas of health care delivery, and bridges over these gaps are frequently developed at the sharp end of practice as people notice that certain tasks are not being done or messages are not getting through. While some bridges may be strong and robust, others may be fragile and vulnerable to minor changes in the system, people leaving the department or efforts to increase efficiency that remove free time (which may be used for informal social activities that contribute to safety). Identifying the knowledge gaps between groups and how these are currently bridged and worked around within each department would appear to be a crucial step in the formal and informal assessment of departmental safe practice. In both of the departments studied here, the crucial role played by the senior nurses would appear to be one area in which a concern for potential gaps may be warranted. When these actors leave the network, a great number of ties between people may be lost. Actions to cope with this could be for the senior nurses themselves to seek to devolve some of their intergroup bridging tasks to other nurse team leaders and making sure successors are fully briefed and socialized within the department before their departure.

The contribution of these informal networks is clearly developed in research and theory related to communities of practice (Lave and Wenger 1991). Communities of practice depict the situated elements of interaction, knowledge sharing and learning that are dependent on mutual engagement and joint enterprise within the workplace, rather than through abstract, codified or externalized activities or process. Central to the concept is that learning occurs as workers are socialized into the routines of work, everyday know-how and shared identities through active participation in the workplace communities, especially as they move from the periphery as a novice to the centre as a fully-fledged member of the community. These ideas help us to understand the significance of knowledge sharing networks, as clinicians working together on a day-to-day basis acquire reciprocal understandings, collaborative styles of work and hence strong working relations. These ideas suggest that problem-solving and learning occurs often without formal acknowledgement or reliance upon management intervention. This is not to say however, that such communities or networks will always be orientated to patient safety, and they may indeed continue to hoard knowledge and stifle needed safety improvements. Equally, we do not suggest that more formal and managed systems of learning should be disregarded in favour of these informal networks. It is worth making explicit therefore how these practice networks have the potential to both contour and confound data collected through formal learning and reporting systems. Practice networks may influence which incidents or activities become common knowledge throughout the department and are deemed significant and requiring of management attention. For example, incidents that are seen as recurring problems are far more likely to be reported, whereas those that are seen as one-offs may be glossed over. Therefore, what is shared informally may affect what is reported formally. That being said, it is still important to share knowledge beyond the immediate clinical environment or network, so as to garner wider lessons and learning opportunities. Our conclusion therefore is that we should not disregard these informal networks of communication or their potential contribution to patient safety, but we should work to find ways in which they can be better harnessed along with more formal learning systems, so as to promote more robust and clinically relevant safety improvements.

References

AHRQ. 2001. *Making Health Care Safer: A Critical Analysis of Patient Safety Practices*. Agency for Healthcare Research and Quality.

Birleson, P. 1998. Learning organizations: an unsuitable model for improving mental health services? *Australian and New Zealand Journal of Psychiatry* 32, 214–222.

Blok, A. 1973 Coalitions in Sicilian peasant society. In Boissevain, J. and Mitchell, J. C. (eds) *Network Analysis: Studies in Human Interaction*. New York: Mouton Publications, 155–166.

Bontis, N. and Sorenko, A. 2009. Longitudinal knowledge strategising in a long term health care organization. *International Journal of Technology Management* 47(3), 276–297.

Borgatti, S. P. and Cross, R. 2003. A relational view of information seeking and learning in social networks. *Management Science* 49(4), 432–445.

Braithwaite, J., Runciman, W. B. and Merry, A. F. 2009. Towards safer, better health care: harnessing the natural properties of complex sociotechnical systems. *Quality and Safety in Health Care* 18, 37–41.

Burt, R. S. 1982. *Toward a Structural Theory of Action: Network Models of Social Structure, Perception, and Action Quantitative Studies in Social Relations.* New York: Academic Press.

Catchpole, K. R., Giddings, A. E. B., Wilkinson, M., Hirst, G., Dale, T. and de Leval, M. R. 2007. Improving patient safety by identifying latent failures in successful operations. *Surgery* 142(1), 102–110.

Chang, A., Schyve, P. M., Croteau, R. J., O'Leary, D. S. and Loeb, J. L. 2005. Patient safety event taxonomy: a standardized terminology and classification schema for near misses and adverse events. *International Journal for Quality in Health Care* 17(2), 95–105.

Coiera, E. and Tombs, V. 1998. Communication behaviours in a hospital setting: an observational study. *British Medical Journal* 316(7132), 673–676.

Coiera, E., Jayasuriya, R. A., Hardy, J., Bannan, A. and Thorpe, M. E. C. 2002. Communication loads on clinical staff in the emergency department. *Medical Journal of Australia* 176(9), 415–418.

Cook, R. L., Render, M. and Woods, D. D. 2000. Gaps in the continuity of care and progress on patient safety. *British Medical Journal* 320(7327), 791–782.

Cott, C. 1997. We decide, you carry it out: a social network analysis of multidisciplinary long-term care teams. *Social Science and Medicine* 45(9), 1411–1421.

Creswick, N., Westbrook, J. L. and Braithwaite, J. 2010. Understanding communication networks in the emergency department. *BMC Health Services Research* 9(247), available from http://www.biomedcentral.com/1472-6963/9/247.

Currie, G. and Suhomlinova, O. 2006. The impact of institutional forces upon knowledge sharing in the UK NHS: the triumph of professional power and the inconsistency of policy. *Public Administration* 84(1), 1–30.

Finn, R., Learmonth, M. and Reedy, P. 2010. Some unintended effects of teamwork in health care. *Social Science and Medicine* 70(8), 1148–1154.

Firth-Cozens, J. 2001. Cultures for improving patient safety through learning: the role of teamwork. *Quality in Health Care* 10(2), 26–31.

Granovetter, M. 1973. The strength of weak ties. *American Journal of Sociology* 78, 1360–1380.

Helmreich, R. L. 2000. On error management: lessons from aviation. *British Medical Journal* 320(7237), 781–789.

Hudson, R. 2004. Analysing network partnerships. *Public Management Review* 6(1), 75–79.

Kaushal, R., Shojania, K. G. and Bates, D. W. 2003. Effects of computerized physician order entry and clinical decision support systems on medication safety: a systematic review. *Archives of Internal Medicine* 163, 1409–1416.

Kennedy, I. 2001. *Bristol Royal Infirmary Inquiry Report.* London: TSO.

Lave, J. and Wenger, E. 1991. *Situated Learning: Legitimate Peripheral Participation.* Cambridge University Press.

Lawton, R. and Parker, D. 2002. Barriers to incident reporting in a health care system. *Quality and Safety in Health Care* 11, 15–18.

Lazarsfeld, P. F. and Merton, R. K. 1954. Friendship as social process: a substantive and methodological analysis. In: Berger M., Abel, T. and Nostrand, V. (eds) *Freedom and Control in Modern Society*. New York: Questia, 18–67.

Levin, D. Z. and Cross, R. 2004. The strength of weak ties you can trust: the mediating role of trust in effective knowledge transfer. *Management Science* 50(11), 1477–1490.

Lewis, K., Kaufman, J., Gonzalez, M., Wimmer, A. and Christakis, N. 2008. Tastes, ties, and time: a new social network dataset using facebook.com. *Social Networks* 30(4), 330–342.

Lorenz, E. H. 1989. Neither friends nor strangers: information networks of subcontracting in French industry. In: Gambretta, D. *Trust: Making and Breaking of Cooperative Relations*. Oxford: Basil Blackwell, 194–210.

March, J. G. and Simon, H. A. 1958. *Organizations*. Chichester: John Wiley and Sons.

Menjivar, C. 1995. Kinship networks among immigrants: lessons from a qualitative comparative approach. *International Journal of Comparative Sociology* 36(3–4), 219–232.

National Patient Safety Agency. 2003. *Annual Report*. London: National Patient Safety Agency.

Neale, G., Woloshynowych, M. and Vincent, C. 2001. Exploring the causes of adverse events in NHS hospital practice. *Journal of the Royal Society of Medicine* 94(7), 322–330.

Putnam, R. D. 1995. Bowling alone: America's declining social capital. *Journal of Democracy* 6(1), 65–78.

Rice, R. E. and Aydin, C. 1991. Attitudes towards new organizational technology: network proximity as a mechanism for social information processing. *Administrative Science Quarterly* 36, 219–244.

Rosenthal, M. M. (1995) *The Incompetent Doctor: Behind Closed Doors*. Buckingham: Open University Press.

Scott, J., Tallia, A., Crosson, J. C., Orzano, A. J., Stroebel, C., DiCicco-Bloom, B., O'Malley, D., Shaw, E. and Crabtree, B. 2005. Social network analysis as an analytic tool for interaction patterns in primary care practices. *Annals of Family Medicine* 3(5), 443–448.

Scott, J. P. 2000. *Social Network Analysis: A Handbook*. London: Sage.

Senge, P. M. 1996. Leading learning organizations. *Training and Development* 50, 36–37.

Tagliaventi, M. R. and Mattarelli, E. M. 2006. The role of networks of practice, value sharing and operational proximity in knowledge flows between professional groups. *Human Relations* 3, 291–391.

Vincent, C., Benn, J. and Hanna, G. B. 2010. High reliability in health care. *British Medical Journal* 340, c84.

Warde, A., Tampubolon, G. and Savage, M. 2005. Recreation, informal social networks and social capital. *Journal of Leisure Research* 37(4), 402–425.

Waring, J. 2005. Beyond blame: the cultural barriers to medical incident reporting. *Social Science and Medicine* 60, 1927–1935.

Waring, J., McDonald, R. and Harrison, S. 2007. Complexity and safety: inter-departmental relationships as a threat to patient safety in the operating department. *Journal of Health, Organization and Management* 20(3), 227–242.

Wasserman, S. and Faust, K. 1994. *Social Network Analysis*. Cambridge: Cambridge University Press.

Weick, K. E. and Sutcliffe, K M. 2001. *Managing the Unexpected: Assuring High Performance in an Age of Complexity*. San Francisco: Jossey-Bass.

West, E., Barron, D. N., Dowsett, J. and Newton, J. N. 1999. Hierarchies and cliques in the social networks of health care professionals: implications for the design of dissemination strategies. *Social Science and Medicine* 48(5), 633–646.

Williams, P. 2002. The competent boundary spanner. *Public Administration* 80, 103–124.

Wilson, K. A., Burke, C. S., Priest, H. A. and Salas, E. 2005. Promoting health care safety through training high reliability teams. *Quality and Safety in Health Care* 14, 303–309.

PART 5
Learning

Chapter 9

Challenges to Learning from Clinical Adverse Events:
A Study of Root Cause Analysis in Practice

Jeanne Mengis and Davide Nicolini

Hospitals rarely learn from failure. This is especially true for the many no-harm, or near miss incidents that occur on a daily basis (Weick and Sutcliffe 2003, Wu et al. 2003, Edmondson 2004). Two arguments are often put forward when explaining this phenomenon. On the one hand, the organization of work in hospitals is shown to favour quick fixes and work-arounds rather than systematic analysis (Tucker and Edmondson 2003, Waring et al. 2007). Highly pressured nurses, for instance, spend around 15 per cent of their time coping with system failures, but deal with these issues mainly through first order problem solving without addressing the underlying causes of the problems (Edmondson 2004). On the other hand, learning from incidents is hampered because the culture between health care providers and within medicine more generally does not incite the admission of error. A very committing context (Weick and Sutcliffe 2003), a 'blame culture' (Nieva and Sorra 2003, Singer et al. 2003), and a lack of psychological safety (Tucker and Edmondson 2003) not only lead to under-reporting of incidents (Waring 2005), but also lead to cover-up strategies, justifications of inadequate performance (Weick and Sutcliffe 2003), and interpersonal situations where people refrain from speaking up about difficult issues or asking questions (Uhlig et al. 2002, Edmondson 2004) . These issues run counter to the aspirations of learning and ultimately threaten patient safety.

Health care institutions across the world have adopted structured investigation procedures, namely root cause analysis (RCA) to address these challenges and foster organizational learning (Department of Health 2001, Department of Veteran Affairs 2008). RCA is the umbrella term to describe a series of methodologies and tools for the retrospective and structured investigation of adverse incidents, near misses and sentinel events (Wald and Shojania 2001). It offers concrete tools for doing more thorough analyses of safety events and thus challenges simple explanations and counters the barriers to learning mentioned above (Amo 1998, Bagian et al. 2002). It can also facilitate a more open safety culture (Leape et al. 1998, Department of Health 2001, Bagian et al. 2002, Kuhn and Youngberg 2002). Carroll et al. (2002) found, for example, that in practice RCA instills doubt and a questioning attitude towards existing assumptions and working practices, which leads to a more open culture where information could be shared more easily across boundaries. In other words, RCA provides the opportunity for clinical staff to step back from their everyday work, to become aware of their own and others' practices, and identify opportunities for learning and change through a structured reflection-on-action process (Schön 1983, Rich and Parker 1995).

Although RCA promises to inform learning in the aftermath of clinical adverse events, we know very little about its effectiveness in the health care context and the challenges of implementing it in daily activity (Wallace 2006, Iedema et al. 2008, Wu et al. 2008). In this chapter, we report the results of an in-depth ethnographic study of the application of RCA in two large hospitals within the English National Health Service (NHS). The aim of the study was to investigate how RCA practices and procedures are undertaken with the intention of identifying the barriers to successful learning and recommendations for service development. The chapter is organized as follows. We start by briefly describing the vision of RCA as outlined in the literature and policy and discuss the perspective of organizational learning that this approach reflects. We then describe the results of our study and highlight the major challenges of implementing RCA on the ground. Finally, we will discuss some of the implications these challenges have for organizational learning. Our chapter complements Chapter 7 in this volume from Waring and Currie who discuss how the long-standing tensions between health professions and service managers can inhibit the reporting of clinical incidents. Not only the reporting, but also the investigation of incidents is faced with a variety of pragmatic problems.

Root Cause Analysis in Health care

RCA is a family of approaches for investigating and engendering learning that have strong links with systems engineering and human factors, which were originally developed to analyse industrial incidents (Carroll 1998, Andersen and Fagerhaug 2000). In line with the human factors approach, RCA directs analytical attention away from 'active' human errors to the 'latent' or systemic factors, and corresponding 'error chains' that condition, enable or exacerbate the potential for active error (Reason 2000).

Like the American and Australian health care systems, the English NHS endorsed RCA as the main tool for incident investigation in 2000 when it became mandatory for all incidents leading to permanent injury or death to be investigated in this way. Following the creation of the National Patient Safety Agency (NPSA) in 2002, more than 8000 NHS staff have been trained in RCA (Wallace 2006), and the approach was promoted more widely as the primary method for organizational learning. Although the NPSA did not mandate a particular process, its training highlighted the template outlined in the 'London Protocol' (Vincent et al. 1998). Investigations should be undertaken by a small operational team; team members should agree the appropriate terms of reference and methods for gathering evidence; team members should be involved in the processes of interrogating, analysing and discussing evidence following various RCA tools; and that team members should participate in the drafting of recommendations for service improvements. In terms of process, when a reported incident is deemed serious enough to warrant an investigation, the necessary data and individual 'witness' statements are collected and a team of experts convened to review the data and generate learning. The role of this team is to analyse information, find out what happened, and develop recommendations that are disseminated within the organization to be implemented.

There is a broad consensus that RCA is a 'toolbox' of up to 40 techniques, rather than a single method for reviewing and analysing collected evidence (Andersen and Fagerhaug 2000, Woloshynowych et al. 2005). Of these, the NPSA (2004) promoted a variety to be used across the investigatory stage, primarily for analysing data and interpreting results. In particular, the team is encouraged to use 'barrier analysis, brainstorming, brain writing, change analysis, five whys, narrative chronology, nominal group technique, tabular timeline, time person grid, and simple timeline' (NPSA, 2004). These tools, in combination with an easy to follow, orderly sequence of procedural steps promises to identify the true cause(s) of a problem and the actions necessary to eliminate it.

Learning through Root Cause Analysis?

RCA has been developed from the human factors approach, system engineering and total quality management (Leape et al. 1998, Bagian et al. 2002, Vincent 2003). Whilst it does not draw on an explicit theory of organizational learning, several of its characteristics appear promising for promoting learning. It provides a 'space' for 'structured reflection' amongst a multidisciplinary 'team' (Baker et al. 2003) and encourages reflective practice more generally by developing a safety-sensitive perspective through which health care professionals can reflect on their work (Schön 1983). The dynamic formation of RCA teams increases the number of people involved first-hand in the management of clinical incidents, which can contribute to a stronger commitment to safe practice (Uhlig et al. 2002).

In spite of these potential benefits, we argue that RCA is a problematic approach because it reflects a problem-driven view of organizational learning (Gherardi 1999, Scarbrough and Swan 2008). This view suggests that learning is achieved through solving a concrete problem. These have to be investigated and understood rationally and then countermeasures need to be put in place, which address the cause(s) of the problem. Thus learning is mainly viewed as a cognitive, rational and step-wise process (Gherardi 1999). For example, RCA involves tools to collect and analyse data in the belief that once the right service improvements are identified, they will be implemented without difficulty and safer practices will automatically follow. A second premise of the problem-driven view of learning is that learning is achieved mainly through continuously updating and correcting suboptimal practices through incident reporting and implementing action plans

(Gherardi 1999). This involves a non-problematic use of written records and files (that is incident forms), which are treated as 'evidence'. Finally, learning is seen as a homogeneous product of experience, where a learning initiative has a directly identifiable and measurable outcome (Gherardi 1999). Table 9.1 juxtaposes Gherardi's (1999) description of problem-driven learning with the model of RCA as articulated in health policies (Department of Health 2001, NPSA 2004).

Table 9.1   The process of incident investigation as an example of problem-driven learning

Process description of 'problem-driven' learning (Gherardi 1999: 108)	Process description of RCA (Department of Health 2001: 31)
'The processes involved in learning are: 1. The observation of relevant instances and the maintenance of a record or a memory of them; 2. The comparison of this memory with some desired outcome; 3. The drawing of conclusions from the comparison; 4. The feeding back of these conclusions to a point where they can influence future performance.'	'There are five components of any investigation: 1. Collect evidence about what happened; 2. Assemble and consider the evidence; 3. Compare the findings with relevant standards, protocols or guidelines, whether national or local, to establish the facts, draw conclusions about causation and make recommendations for action to minimize risk; 4. Draw up an improvement strategy with prioritized actions, responsibilities, timescales and strategies for measuring the effectiveness of actions; 5. Implement the improvement strategy and track progress, including the effectiveness of actions.'

Whilst RCA and the problem-driven approach suggest that learning and change occur through a rational and linear process, our argument is that the approach does not take into account the *organizing* of learning. Learning and change are situated and embedded in practice and learning initiatives meet – in view also of the organizational entanglements and political dimension of learning (see Chapter 7 this volume) – a variety of practical challenges. Our research surfaces the challenges that arise when implementing a problem-driven approach such as RCA and explores the implications for organizational learning.

Methods

The research followed in the ethnographic tradition (Fetterman 1998), which is now well-established in the field of patient safety research (Finn and Waring

2006). The benefit of ethnography is that it provides the opportunity to observe first-hand how patient safety events transpire, are communicated and analysed. In particular, it allows research to understand how RCA activities are arranged and undertaken, to consider how they reflect or indeed break with established customs and ways of working, and to explore the actual and potential contributions to organizational learning.

The study was undertaken over 12 months in two English NHS Trusts located in different regions. Trust A was a medium-sized general hospital with 6000 staff and treating 500,000 patients per year; Trust B was a large teaching hospital with 12,000 staff and treating over one million patients per year. After an initial period of identifying the organizational arrangements within each Trust, the study 'tracked' 10 incident investigations from start to finish. For all cases we observed how the investigation team was formed; how evidence was collected; how RCA tools were used; how error chains and root cause factors were identified; and how recommendations and findings were drafted and disseminated. During this period we conducted 102 ethnographic interviews to clarify events, and completed 34 semi-structured interviews with those involved in the investigations. These interviews centred on the experiences of participating in an investigation, the use of RCA tools, the perceived contributions and barriers to organizational learning. Our findings were analysed by the research team to identify and understand the barriers to using RCA and to determine its contribution to organizational learning.

Challenges Along the RCA Process

Forming the Investigation Team and Gathering Evidence

The formation of a knowledgeable and respected team is integral to undertaking a robust and inclusive investigation and for generating legitimate recommendations for change. Although there are no strict guidelines, teams are typically composed of representatives of the various health care groups contributing to the care of the patient at the centre of the investigation. The formation of this team is challenging. A preliminary obstacle is securing the involvement of those individuals who played a key role in the incident or who have in-depth knowledge of the health care processes related to the incident. This both delayed the investigation and also created frustration among the rest of the team:

> I think the rambling in this meeting had to do with the fact that we did not know certain facts. And we did not know them because the relevant people were not present.
>
> Consultant.

Multiple reasons were mentioned for this absenteeism. Some clinicians avoided participation because they lacked confidence in the usefulness of RCA process, others feared the potential to be 'convicted' or blamed, and others still appeared to be concerned with protecting their interests or reputation. However, many simply could not attend because they experienced 'diary conflicts' or in some cases were no longer employed by the organization. In view of this, risk managers often had to balance between the completeness of the team and the timeliness of the investigation.

Similar challenges were identified in relation to the collection of evidence. During several RCA meetings we observed clinicians or managers frustration about missing, incomplete, or contradictory information which made it difficult to understand the sequence of events and determine the related causes and contributory factors that contextualized an incident:

> There were about four different sheets with different people recording his level of pain over the same time period, none of which matched up. We would have needed the log from the PCA machine, which would have told us how many times he pressed the button in order to get the analgesia.

Consultant/Clinical Director

This quotation highlights a further problem related to the quality of information provided in case notes and statements. Specifically, patient and clinical records, whilst providing detailed diagnostic and treatment information for patient care, often contained insufficient or inappropriate information for the purpose of investigation. In short, this information was compiled for a different purpose and its role in the investigation was complicated by this fact. As such, lead investigators were often required to trawl additional information sources, such as computer systems, staff rotas and maintenance records. Accordingly, evidence often represented a patchwork of information that needed to be carefully weaved together to provide different perspectives of the event. This proved particularly difficult when cases were ambiguous and clinical judgements varied across the various clinical specialties.

Investigators faced several challenges in the early stages of the RCA process, from securing the willing participation of staff, to being confident of the quality of information contained within records and statements and dealing with the ambiguity of clinical 'facts'. This in turn affected the quality of evidence and the accuracy and legitimacy of subsequent analysis and recommendations. In many cases, these initial challenges stem from the fact that the success of RCA investigations depends in part on organizational conditions and a positive safety culture that the tool itself aims at producing.

Conducting the Analysis and Identifying Root Causes

At the centre of all RCA processes was the facilitated 'RCA meeting' involving the whole investigation team. This was the primary setting for communicating and scrutinizing collected evidence, applying RCA tools, identifying error chains and risk factors and developing recommendations. During these meetings, an incident would be reviewed and scrutinized drawing on the prepared timeline and the collected evidence and relevant policy procedures. The various service providers deliberate collectively upon the causes of the incident.

One of the most significant challenges in this process related to the influence of professional status on participation. During the meetings, turn-taking tended to follow a hierarchical pattern with doctors speaking first and most often, senior nurses and managers having some voice, and junior staff speaking only when asked. In many cases, group interaction was dominated by one or two professional or managerial representatives who held (or assumed) greater authority. These difficulties also applied to RCA facilitators who were outwardly presented as leading the investigation by virtue of their formal organizational role in risk management, but who during these meetings were often relegated to a marginal position. In many cases this appeared to result from their clinical background or inexperience which limited their participation and ability to direct interaction. This weak position could be observed, for example, when they repeatedly asked clinicians 'what do you do normally', which signalled their lack of know-how about clinical procedures. Through asking such questions, incidents often got reframed by clinicians as 'outliers' or rare events that were completely anomalous and out of the norm. Consequently, they were presented as infrequent, not related to 'normal' work and therefore not worthy of thorough investigation because only limited learning would follow. This can be seen as the inverse of what Vaughan (1996) and Waring (2005) called the normalization of deviance (that is, incidents are part of the life of hospitals), but interestingly it had the same effect as normalization. 'Normally' procedures were in place and under control, such that incidents did not require further inquiry.

Another significant finding was that most of the investigation teams made few attempts to utilize the available RCA techniques and tools, such as the '5 whys' or 'fishbone' tools, which systematically focus attention to latent factors. Across all incidents the timeline was the only observed method used to map and analyse evidence. The critical question here is whether this derives from a lack of training in the RCA toolkit (Wallace 2006), some form of resistance to their use, or whether these tools do not speak to the nature of the practice they are supposed to investigate. Specifically, the time-orientated style of analysis aligned more closely with clinicians' mindset and mode of work than the tools drawn from the engineering tradition. For instance, temporality is a strong organizer of medical work (that is, diagnosis then treatment), both for individual health care providers in the form of temporal horizons (that is, what to do first and after, what are fixed deadlines, what is urgent?), and for the collective health care team as temporal rhythms (nursing shifts, rounds, drug response time) (Zerubavel 1979, Reddy et al. 2006). While most RCA tools are aimed at providing an atemporal, analytic and oversight or 'helicopter' view of the complex system of care and how it interacts around a safety event, health care practitioners favour tools that help them reconstruct the event in its temporal unfolding and from the perspective of 'being there', as if they extended the present to the past (Ricoeur 1984).

Finally, many potential root causes were discounted during these analysis meetings. For instance, a potential latent risk was identified and discussed by participants, but then discounted or passed over for another factor or series of events. This appeared to happen where the identified factor was deemed too complex and ambiguous, and where it could not be easily resolved through the implementation of a single containable countermeasure. This issue was compounded by the time and resource pressure the analytical teams operated within, which required them to produce quick and tangible results. Accordingly, analysis tended to centre on either the identification of factors that could be easily 'fixed' or the allocation of responsibility (shifting of blame) to organizational groups typically not represented in the process.

Our findings suggest that in practice RCA does not lead to a robust, comprehensive analysis of clinical incidents where root causes and contributory factors are carefully identified and appraised. We observed that there is a clear preference for narrative and temporal accounts and that there is a general orientation towards 'closure' rather than inquiry. The main challenges to analysis were not cognitive, but rather socio-political, psychological and organizational in nature. RCAs were characterized by unequal participation and by resource and time constraints, which orientated analysis towards the generation of tangible, uncomplicated and linear interpretations of risk, and quick, inexpensive and measurable solutions. Policy-makers might question therefore whether the current, mainly cognitive support for doing RCA (that is providing tools for identifying contributory factors) is attuned to the nature of the clinical activity and the challenges faced in the investigation process.

Formulating and Implementing Change

The investigation report is both the end product of the process and the tool through which recommendations are circulated for future implementation. An elaborate set of activities are involved in the production of the report: statements written, timelines developed, RCA meetings documented, causal factors defined and explained and investigation reports formulated. These work practices are all oriented on documentation, accounting and control. The dealings with these and the production of the final report seemed, at times, to become an 'end in itself' without necessarily contributing to learning or change.

Elaborating upon this view, the investigation report occupies a central role in the RCA process because it serves to demonstrate, and verify that all necessary procedures and policies have been followed. Brown (2000) argued similarly, in his analysis of public inquiries, that through presenting an acceptable interpretation of events, investigation reports work to re-establish organizational legitimacy, which in our case is the legitimacy of the Trusts or clinical departments. As such, it is designed to create reassurance and confidence both in the process and the organization. We observed, for example, that the dissent and conflict often observed in RCA meetings was largely left out of the reports and that the language used rarely gave a sense of the uncertainty or controversy the investigation team experienced in identifying root causes. The reports therefore provide an uncontested, non-ambiguous review of the 'facts'. For instance, accounts and statements that were framed with 'I do believe' or 'I cannot clearly remember' were presented in the report as ascertained facts lacking any additional qualifier and being mainly written in the passive tense. Through these means, the report reinstalled reassurance where the incident had created ambiguity, if not anxiety (Brown 2000). Finally, reassurance was achieved also by narrating the incident as a linear sequence of events. The sequencing of events is an important source of sense making (Ricoeur 1984, Weick 1995) as it suggests that what follows is caused by what preceded (Patriotta 2003). Yet the very linear account often neglected the complex details of how the various latent factors related or combined.

This could be further seen in the way report recommendations were constructed to produce a convincing, receivable and workable action plan, which compounded the tendency to discuss issues in terms of available solutions, rather than 'root causes'. The causal factors identified were thus phrased in terms of: 'what would have helped here...', or 'what we do in obstetrics in such occasions is to...'. Recommendations were therefore limited by a lack of attention to the complexity of causal factors and depth of analysis. In turn, this meant that change centred on small improvements or interventions that could be delivered at a local, departmental level. This included disciplinary action or additional training for staff, but neglected attention to wider organizational improvements that might involve more substantial resource implications, which were seen as 'beyond the gift' of the investigation team. The reports were also driven to produce change that could be easily delivered and audited at the local level, with clear expectations of goals and targets.

Finally, and somewhat surprisingly, we found no evidence that the investigation teams or Trusts had a coherent orientation towards managing the change process following the production of recommendations. Although risk managers had received training and perfected their skills in diagnosing patient safety problems, they were totally unprepared to address the challenges of turning recommendations into sustainable service transformation. When action plans were followed through and changes were introduced in clinical practice, it was less than certain that these would persist over time. This is a particular challenge in view of the high turnover of staff as outlined by a ward manager of the emergency department:

> What you implement can be very straightforward ... That would be as simple as sending a memo out, but the making sure this is still happening in a year's

time, that's what is challenging ... We have junior doctors turning over every
four months, ... having to educate them on all the policies and protocols in the
department is quite challenging.

Ward manager

Overall, the translation of the action plans into the practice was a challenging
and complex activity. In short, incident investigations were de-coupled from
practice, and were poorly reconciled with the intricacies of the practical, material
and temporal arrangements of delivering and improving health care service.
However, the issue of how to facilitate the change process, how to address the
likely resistances to change and how to fit the changes needed to prevent the
reoccurrence of incidents with competing agendas and initiatives were scarcely
if ever considered.

Dealing with Emotions and Overcoming a Culture of Blame

Most of the literature on RCA presents the process as a rational and technical
endeavour. Little or no attention is paid to the role of emotions such as anxiety, fear
and shame in the different stages of the RCA process. Our study found, however,
that emotions affect the RCA process in at least three ways.

First, the RCA process, especially the RCA meeting, is a highly emotional
process. People involved in incidents often develop an unspoken sense of guilt
that significantly increases stress at work. We observed a case, for example,
where a member of staff involved in a fatal incident was so troubled about
her responsibility that she fell sick for several weeks in the aftermath. When
investigation teams were composed of staff directly involved in the incident, one
benefit of the RCA process was that it helped these people come to terms with their
emotions through an elaboration of mourning (Grindberg 1964). Specifically, the
RCA meeting offered a chance to collectively repair the social sense of trust in
the existing work procedures and arrangements, a necessary condition for people
to function in human organisations. Yet, while some individual RCA facilitators
were good at building up a trusting and appreciative atmosphere, others were less
so. In addition, the stated aim of RCA meetings (to analyse the relevant evidence
and identify the root cause of an incident) did not legitimize emotions, which were
thus often poorly managed. The result was meetings where discussion failed to
progress and learning suffered.

Second, blame and fear of being blamed are still present during the RCA
process. While the idea of 'no blame' is at the core of current approaches to
learning from adverse events (Barach and Small 2000, Vince and Saleem 2004),
it remains a distant ideal. Consider the following quote from an interview with a
senior house officer:

even in the meeting I did hear that: 'oh, this nurse who did this has been told about this, has done retraining'. Well, if it's a no-blame culture and someone is not really wrong, then why are we trying to witch hunt different people? I don't think there is a no-blame culture. I think that RCAs are looking for fault.

Senior House Officer

Throughout the RCA processes, blame remained in circulation, yet by imposing a strict politically correct way of speaking, blaming takes place in a less open form and is swept under the proverbial carpet. In fact, the no-blame discourse and failure to take into account the anxiety of being accused of failure creates a number of 'un-discussables'. We observed, for example, how questions of responsibility and blame often featured in the informal meetings and conversations that occurred outside the formal RCA processes. The prevailing no-blame edict therefore merely served to conceal or displace blame within the official investigations.

Third, organizational pressures and a fear of control are also present during RCA processes. We found that RCA was often perceived as a form of control stemming from the 'centre', often exacerbated by the close links between the central risk management functions of each hospital and the claims and complaints office. This vicinity adds to the perception that RCA is almost a legal investigation with a concern with culpability and discipline. When this applies, RCA investigators are interpreted and regarded by clinical representatives as intruders and potential threats instead of partners in the change effort. This lack of psychological safety (Edmondson 1999, Tucker and Edmondson 2003) in turn negatively affects the quality of the process and the capacity to produce usable results.

Bounded Learning

One of the assumptions behind the use of RCA is that it enables health care professionals to shed light on the intricacies of the work practices, people and objects of their hospital through a system-sensitive analysis of a single incident. In others, the single event can be used to draw out wider lesson for more general and systemic service improvement. When observing RCA meetings, however, we could see that participants tried to draw narrow boundaries of where the system ended and where change should occur. In one occasion, for example, the discussion of an incident centred on the quality of medical record keeping. The obstetrician exclaimed: 'Let's not go there, that's another jar of worms'. Similar comments were made throughout the RCA meeting where participants actively tried to keep the discussion tightly bound to the local level. It was not only the analysis of the problem that was limited to the local level, but also the scope of the proposed solutions. In both hospitals, questions of resources and cost often framed how potential solutions were discussed and presented. A risk officer commented as follows: 'We can't propose changes that cost a lot. Otherwise, we would need a business case. That is why we usually suggest only small adjustments.'

RCA's aspiration to analyse a system through a local event turns back on itself so that 'system', 'causes' and 'solutions' are constructed and limited to the local, not the system. This extends what Iedema et al. (2006a: 1612) called the 'micro-sociology of clinical failure' where clinicians are 'disabled from intervening in matters superordinate to clinical treatment' (that is resource allocation). Moreover, RCA makes clinicians limit their focus on only those aspects of clinical treatment which can be locally rearranged and require very limited resources. One clinical director described this issue of micro-managing problems through single incidents as follows:

> There are major systems issues in the trust that are raised time, and time, and time again. It needs a large-scale strategic manoeuvre to put it back together and change things. We've got major problems in this Trust with identifying where patients are, who's looking after them, having patients on the wrong wards ... You get a sense that the problems are just ongoing and that there's no coordinated approach to dealing with them.

Clinical Director

One way to move from the micro perspective of single incidents to a more system-level perspective is to reflect upon patterns and trends of similar incidents. Although we found several weekly departmental, audit and review meetings within both hospitals, including dedicated incident review meetings, these again tended to be limited to the more local issues related to individual patient safety events; as is shown in the following excerpt from the field notes.

> K. [the ward manager from ED] meets with M. [the clinical risk officer] for their weekly Clinical Adverse Event meeting. She tells the number of the patient, scans through the description of the incident as it is put in the report and then M. tells her what the status of the incident is: 'Ohh, that's closed', or: 'I've to look into this one'. They have a brief conversation on one of the incidents. M says: 'Now, this is what H. said. In radiology they have a discrepancy with you.' K. replies: 'Ok, I'll talk to her' They then move on to the next incidents. M. looks at one incident form and K. comments: 'This one is medical, but does not go to M. It goes to the divisional medical director'.

In this brief interaction it is striking that despite the large amount of incidents the two officers reviewed – 35 new incidents were discussed in that particular meeting – they stuck to an individual discussion of each individual case and did not discuss patterns of similar incidents conjointly. Only occasionally did they pause to note recurring patterns using expressions such as: 'they all happen together', 'it's another one of those', or 'it's the same old story'. But even in such cases, this did not lead to a more systematic analysis. At the most, they would tell an anecdote of a similar incident that occurred recently, such as 'this reminds me of another case we had recently'.

Things are slightly different when a series of similar and usually major or fatal incidents occur within a short time frame. In these rare cases, support from senior management leads to a more speedy investigation. In addition, there is an expectation that recommendations for change can be more substantial and costly. One point in case was the occurrence of three similar major incidents within a time frame of five months, where three patients died because of delayed treatment within the same department. Although the three cases were analysed independently, by the time of the third incident a major review was enacted and a 24/7 emergency call service introduced to prevent similar events. One consultant described how they would not 'wait for a pattern of the same incident', and if similar situations present again they are now able to 'flag it' and 'act on it straight away'. He added: 'It is not easy to receive the money for a 24/7 on call service. But with three similar incidents in a row, nobody can argue against it.' A pattern of similar incidents can therefore add strength and urgency to the implementation of more substantial and expensive changes, despite the focus of analysis often remaining at the level of the single incident.

Conclusions

Although RCA provides a powerful tool for informing learning, its use in the health care context remains problematic. Our study in two English NHS hospitals shows that the practice of RCA meets serious challenges and that we have to question its capability to first, produce more thorough, system-oriented analyses and second to overcome a culture of blame.

Regarding the first, clear challenges are found with the formation of the investigation team, the gathering of evidence, the analysis of data and the formulation and implementation of service improvements. Together these show that far from being a rational and linear process of learning, it is a complex, nested, conflictive, recursive and negotiated social process. RCA, with its problem-driven view on learning (Gherardi 1999), suggests that such difficulties are mainly technical and, accordingly, proposes tools and procedures to address these analytical and cognitive challenges. On the contrary, our study suggests that the challenges in dealing with incidents are largely political, organizational and emotional in nature. The reluctance to identify 'root' causes stems not from analytical difficulty, but from the need to develop feasible, measurable and controllable solutions that can provide, within a short timeframe, reassurance and legitimacy. This transforms the objective of RCA from systemic learning to the production of a neat, convincing and extensive report.

We also suggest that blame, fear and anxiety still permeate the investigation process. Moreover, RCA becomes a device to allocate rationally and legitimately individual or departmental responsibility for patient safety events. By officially banning blame and imposing a politically correct way of reflecting on incidents, blaming has been pushed underground, thereby making it less visible and more difficult to manage. At the same time, RCA's technical and almost scientific language and tools combined with its highly structured approach do not provide an ideal setting for health care providers to mourn and emotionally come to terms with a tragic incident.

Our findings complement previous research, especially studies of RCA conducted in the UK and Australia (Iedema et al. 2006b, Wu et al. 2008). These highlight how resource and time constraints and a lack of expertise can hinder investigation processes and constrain service improvement. Our findings suggest, however, that the challenges of undertaking RCA are more closely linked to its focus on technical matters, on linear and rational processes, and on single incidents, rather than on more socio-cultural, complex, recursive and systemic incidents (vis-à-vis a more epidemiological perspective). Our study indicates that a problem-driven view of organizational learning, which lies at the heart of RCA, has serious consequences for learning on the ground. Specifically, by assuming that learning can be managed as a cognitive, linear process, in practice RCA becomes fixated with facilitating and symbolically creating and maintaining this prescribed process. It does not, however, lend itself to ensuring that learning, especially learning that emerges from and is situated within the RCA process, leads to service improvement. Furthermore, by suggesting that learning is a homogeneous product, action plans tend to focus on the production of discrete, measurable outcomes, which result in local micro-changes. On the other hand, less direct and explicit changes that emanate from RCA, such as an improved relationship between clinical departments or the increased awareness of another team's work, are not appreciated as they are not directly part of the prescribed RCA process. Finally, the outcomes of RCA, such as the statements, the timeline and the investigation report, are used in a non-problematic way, as 'evidence' that can inform the policy-making and the management of a hospital. Instead, our study has shown that all the products of RCA are carefully constructed following the logics and interests of the organization.

In terms of recommendation for practice, our findings suggest that in order to promote learning from clinical incidents, more attention needs to be paid to the organizational, political and emotional processes of learning in health care organizations. This implies, more specifically, that policy-makers need to be more careful in linking multiple, potentially conflicting interests to specific initiatives, such as RCA. An approach or tool, appropriate for (re-)establishing legitimacy and circumventing litigation is not likely to also promote organizational learning. Rather than merely focusing on documentation and control, health care organizations should actively promote the use of less formalized learning processes such as mentoring systems, reflection, sharing between and across professional peers and communities of practice (Adler et al. 2008). These mechanism are useful both for establishing ongoing reflection on practice, but also for strengthening personal relationships and providing the necessary psychological safety for dealing with clinical incidents (Edmondson 1999). Organizations should also explore new instruments such as video-based reflection (Iedema et al. 2009) which can be used to trigger reflection practices that are not necessarily centred on clinical incidents and errors and focus instead on the existing sources of resilience of the organization. Such initiatives do not counter, but can complement RCA as organizational learning is stem from a coordinated set of loosely coupled initiatives rather than one, top-down, single initiative.

References

Adler, P. S., Kwon, S. W. and Heckscher, C. 2008. Professional work: the emergence of collaborative community, *Organization Science*, 19(2), 359–376.

Amo, M. 1998. Root cause analysis. A tool for understanding why accidents occur, *Balance (Alexandria, Va.)*, 2(5), 12.

Andersen, B. and Fagerhaug, T. 2000. *Root Cause Analysis: Simplified Tools and Techniques*, Milwaukee: ASQ Quality Press.

Bagian, J. P., Gosbee, J., Lee, C. Z., Williams, L., McKnight, S. D. and Mannos, D. M. 2002. The Veterans Affairs root cause analysis system in action, *Joint Commission Journal on Quality and Patient Safety*, 28(10), 531–545.

Baker, D. P., Gustafson, S., Beaubien, J., Salas, E. and Barach, P. 2003. *Medical Teamwork and Patient Safety: The Evidence-based Relation*, Rockville, MD: Center for Quality Improvement and Patient Safety Agency for Healthcare Research & Quality.

Barach, P. and Small, S. D. 2000. Reporting and preventing medical mishaps: lessons from non-medical near miss reporting systems, *British Medical Journal*, 320, 759–763.

Brown, A. D. 2000. Making sense of inquiry sensemaking, *Journal of Management Studies*, 37(1), 45–75.

Carroll, J. 1998. Organizational learning activities in high-hazard industries: the logics underlying self-analysis, *Journal of Management Studies*, 35(6), 699–717.

Carroll, J. S., Rudolph, J. W. and Hatakenaka, S. 2002. Lessons learned from non-medical industries: root cause analysis as culture change at a chemical plant, *Quality Safety Health Care*, 11, 266–269.

Department of Health. 2001. *Doing Less Harm. Improving the Safety and Quality of Care through Reporting, Analysing and Learning from Adverse Incidents Involving NHS Patients – Key Requirements for Health Care Providers*, London: Department of Health.

Department of Veteran Affairs. 2008. *VHA National Patient Safety Improvement Handbook*, Washington: Department of Veteran Affairs, Veterans Health Administration.

Edmondson, A. 1999. Psychological safety and learning behavior in work teams, *Administrative Science Quarterly*, 44(2), 350–383.

Edmondson, A. C. 2004. Learning from failure in health care: frequent opportunities, pervasive barriers, *Quality of Safety in Health Care*, 13, ii3–ii9.

Fetterman, D. 1998. *Ethnography: Step by Step*, 2nd ed., Thousand Oaks: Sage.

Finn, R. and Waring, J. 2006. Ethnographic methods in patient safety. In: *Patient Safety: Research into Practice*, K. Walshe and R. Boaden (eds). Maidenhead (UK): Open University Press, 161–172.

Gherardi, S. 1999. Learning as problem-driven or learning in the face of mystery? *Organization Studies*, 20(1), 101–123.

Grindberg, L. 1964. Two kings of guilt – their relations with normal and pathological aspects of morning, *The International Journal of Psychoanalysis*, 45, 366–371.

Iedema, R., Jorm, C., Long, D., Braithwaite, J., Travaglia, J. and Westbrook, M. 2006a. Turning the medical gaze in upon itself: root cause analysis and the investigation of clinical error, *Social Science and Medicine*, 62, 1605–1615.

Iedema, R., Jorm, C., Braithwaite, J., Travaglia, J. and Lum, M. 2006b. A root cause analysis of clinical error: confronting the disjunction between formal rules and situated clinical activity, *Social Science and Medicine*, 63(5), 1201–1212.

Iedema, R., Jorm, C. and Braithwaite, J. 2008. Managing the scope and impact of root cause analysis recommendations, *Journal of Health Organization and Management*, 22(6), 569–585.

Iedema, R., Merrick, E. T., Rajbhandari, D., Gardo, A., Stirling, A. and Herkes, R. 2009. Viewing the taken-for-granted from under a different aspect: a video-based method in pursuit of patient safety, *International Journal of Multiple Research Approaches*, 3(3), 290–301.

Kuhn, A. M. and Youngberg, B. J. 2002. The need for risk management to evolve to assure a culture of safety, *Quality and Safety in Health Care*, 11(2), 158–162.

Leape, L. L., Woods, D. D., Hatlie, M. J., Kizer, K. W., Schroeder, S. A. and Lundberg, G. D. 1998. Promoting patient safety by preventing medical error, *Journal of the American Medical Association*, 280(16), 1444–1447.

Nieva, V. F. and Sorra, J. 2003. Safety culture assessment: a tool for improving patient safety in health care organizations, *Quality and Safety in Health Care*, 12(suppl 2), ii17–ii23.

NPSA. 2004. *Root Cause Analysis Toolkit*, http://www.msnpsa.nhs.uk/rcatoolkit/course/iindex.htm, accessed March 2011.

Patriotta, G. 2003. Sensemaking on the shop floor: narratives of knowledge in organizations, *Journal of Management Studies*, 40(2), 349–375.

Reason, J. T. 2000. Human error: models and management, *British Medical Journal*, 320, 768–770.

Reddy, M. C., Dourish, P. and Pratt, W. 2006. Temporality in medical work: time also matters, *Computer Supported Cooperative Work*, 15(1), 29–53.

Rich, A. and Parker, D. L. 1995. Reflection and critical incident analysis: ethical and moral implications of their use within nursing and midwifery education, *Journal of Advanced Nursing*, 22(6), 1050–1057.

Ricoeur, P. 1984. *Time and Narrative*, Chicago: University of Chicago Press.

Scarbrough, H. and Swan, J. 2008. Project work as a locus of learning: the journey through practice. In: *Community, Economic Creativity, and Organization*, edited by A. Amin and J. Roberts, Oxford: Oxford University Press, 148–177.

Schön, D. A. 1983. *The Reflective Practitioner: How Professionals Think in Action*, New York: Basic Books.

Singer, S. J., Gaba, D. M., Geppert, J. J., Sinaiko, A. D., Howard, S. K. and Park, K. C. 2003. The culture of safety: results of an organization-wide survey in 15 California hospitals, *Quality and Safety in Health Care*, 12(2), 112–118.

Tucker, A. and Edmondson, A. 2003. Why hospitals don't learn from failures: organizational and psychological dynamics that inhibit system change, *California Management Review*, 45(2), 55–72.

Uhlig, P. N., Brown, J., Nason, A. K., Camelio, A. and Kendall, E. 2002. System innovation: Concord hospital, *Joint Commission Journal on Quality and Patient Safety*, 28(12), 666–672.

Vaughan, D. 1996. *The Challenger Launch Decision: Risky Technology, Culture, And Deviance at NASA*, Chicago: University of Chicago Press.

Vince, R. and Saleem, T. 2004. The impact of caution and blame on organizational learning, *Management Learning*, 133–154.

Vincent, C. 2003. Understanding and responding to adverse events, *New England Journal of Medicine*, 34(11), 1051–1056.

Vincent, C., Taylor-Adams, S. and Stanhope, N. 1998. Framework for analysing risk and safety in clinical medicine, *British Medical Journal*, 316(7138), 1154.

Wald, H. and Shojania, K. 2001. Root cause analysis, *Making Health Care Safer: A Critical Analysis of Patient Safety Practices*, 51.

Wallace, L. 2006. From root causes to safer systems: international comparisons of nationally sponsored health care staff training programmes, *British Medical Journal*, 15(6), 388.

Waring, J. 2005. Beyond blame: cultural barriers to medical incident reporting, *Social Science and Medicine*, 60(9), 1927–1935.

Waring, J., Harrison, S. and McDonald, R. 2007. A culture of safety or coping? Ritualistic behaviours in the operating theatre, *Journal of Health Services Research and Policy*, 12(Suppl. 1), 3–9.

Weick, K. E. 1995. *Sensemaking in Organizations,* Thousand Oaks: Sage.

Weick, K. E. and Sutcliffe, K. M. 2003. Hospitals as cultures of entrapment: a re-analysis of the Bristol Royal Infirmary, *California Management Review*, 45(2), 73–84.

Woloshynowych, M., Rogers, S., Taylor-Adams, S. and Vincent, C. 2005. The investigation and analysis of critical incidents and adverse events in health care, *Health Technology Assessment*, 9(19), 1–158.

Wu, A., Lipshutz, A. and Pronovost, P. 2008. Effectiveness and efficiency of root cause analysis in medicine, *Journal of the American Medical Association*, 299(6), 685.

Wu, A. W., Folkman, S., McPhee, S. J. and Lo, B. 2003. Do house officers learn from their mistakes? *Quality and Safety in Health Care*, 12(3), 221–226.

Zerubavel, E. 1979. *Patterns of Time in Hospital Life: A Sociological Perspective*, Chicago: University of Chicago Press.

Chapter 10

Patient Safety and Clinical Practice Improvement:
The Importance of Reflecting on Real-time, In Situ Care Processes

Rick Iedema

As the last century came to a close, the adverse impact of clinical incidents on patients' well-being had become a prominent concern for policy-makers (Department of Health 2000, Institute of Medicine 2001), a focus of formal investigation among clinicians (Berwick 1998), and a source of unease for the wider public (Meek 2001). While in decades past 'patient safety failures have rarely had consequences for health care organizations or those who lead them' (Walshe and Boaden 2006: 5), those in charge of contemporary health services now have little option but to devise ways to ensure an adequate quality of care and level of safety for patients. Nowadays health care managers are dismissed over clinical safety issues; immense political mileage is made out of health service failures, and governments may lose elections and politicians their jobs. For example, in Australia, the Camden and Campbelltown 'affair' was initiated by whistleblower allegations made by three nurses in relation to concerns for patient care, quality and safety (Van Der Weyden 2004). No fewer than six investigations were conducted (Pain and Lord 2006), calling the initial New South Wales Healthcare Complaints Commissioner's investigation into doubt. In the end, no charges against practitioners were supported and the investigations concluded that the Commissioner's original findings were accurate (Pain and Lord 2006). Nevertheless, and before the investigations were concluded, several managers lost their jobs and the Commissioner was given a summary and public dismissal for a perceived failure on the part of the Commission's investigators to find anyone to be individually accountable (Van Der Weyden 2004).

To contextualize these matters, this chapter begins with an overview of approaches that have targeted patient safety. As I review these approaches, I will highlight their commonalities, especially the way they privilege formalized knowledge such as guidelines, evidence and idealized pathways. The metaphor that best characterizes these approaches is that of 'roll-out of ready-made, best-practice solutions'. In reviewing these approaches, I emphasize that they have produced important results, and that they belong to a paradigm that regards the portability and transferability of formal knowledge as the principal function of patient safety intervention.

The chapter then moves on to a section that describes approaches that belong to a complementary paradigm, whose principal metaphor is not 'knowledge' but 'relating'. In this section I articulate the general parameters and practical achievements of approaches that fall under this second paradigm. I outline the main differences between this complementary paradigm and the first paradigm. The principal difference is that approaches in this second paradigm put an emphasis on experiential depth, contextual specificity and social relationships. This second paradigm acknowledges that people often act under suboptimal circumstances, with incomplete information and answering to competing demands. This means they need to be attentive to the changing contexts and dynamics of their work and to each other. Put differently, they need to anticipate the changing potential for failure (Cook and Woods 1994). I discuss three approaches that capture these aspects of front-line clinical work in some detail: experience-based enquiry, expansive learning and video-reflexive ethnography.

The conclusion of the chapter points to safety requiring clinicians to have access to times and spaces where the complexity of their everyday work and their responses to it can be revisited in a trustful and creative manner. This reflexive practice arises from people together discussing frictions in care and taking account of different stakeholders' interests and perspectives, including those of clinicians, managers, researchers, patients, patients' families, policy-makers and funders. In taking these different perspectives into account, clinicians come to define outcomes, improvements and failures in terms that, instead of privileging their own worldviews, backgrounds and perspectives, are inclusive of others' experiences, questions and perspectives. When this second paradigm comes about, safety is recognized to be contingent upon reflexivity (Iedema 2011), or the adoption of a new structure of attention (Thrift 2004a).

Prevailing Approaches to Promoting Patient Safety

Policy-makers' concerns about the safety and quality of care have resulted in far-reaching reform. While the direction and intensity of health reform differs between nations, it is becoming clear that reform initiatives have begun to affect and inform most levels or strata of health service organizations (Leatherman 2007).

Thus, in the policy and national infrastructure stratum, reform has centred on the development and implementation of nationwide regulation, inspection and accreditation initiatives, alongside improved public reporting of performance. In the macro-managerial stratum of state, area and district health departments, reform has manifested (among other things) in the development of clinical and organizational targets, benchmarks, standards, guidelines and performance indicators. The informating of clinical work that this has entailed serves to make public reporting possible, but it also enhances this second stratum's control over the third: local health services, including hospitals, medical centres and community health services. Among the more prominent consequences for this third stratum are care quality control, new forms of decision support and internal market financing. Finally, in the stratum of health services provision – the clinical front line, health reform has produced more rigorous kinds of peer and performance appraisal, and widespread analysis, formalization and regulation of work processes. In this stratum, we are witnessing not just bureaucratic and scientific authorities imposing rules on how clinical care is to be provided, but also clinical teams systematizing and engaging in problem-solving their own work practices. Seen from a more general perspective, across these four strata the aim is to render clinical care processes more predictable, effective, efficient and safe.

For its part, when the issue of patient safety first came onto the international agenda in the early 1990s, the principal response centred on structuring and redesigning care processes. This was done on the basis of embedding scientific evidence into bureaucratic and technological forcing functions (Norman 1988) which served to channel action. Here, the preoccupation is to create general principles and resources for action that can be 'applied' to and by large populations of clinicians and patients. The implementation of medical protocols and clinical practice guidelines became the cornerstone of patient safety and practice improvement (Lomas et al. 1991, Woolf et al. 1999).

It was soon evident that these principles and resources faced three important challenges. One was that experts at times disagree about how medical or clinical principles are to be written into guidelines and protocols (Steinberg and Luce 2005). Alongside such disagreements, the fact that practice guidelines are not sensitive to the peculiarities of services, processes, situations or patients (McLaughlin 2001) may explain why guidelines and protocols often face local adoption problems (McGlynn et al. 2003). Finally, it is not uncommon that the implementation of new ways of working are accompanied by new errors and lead to new problems (Tenner 1996). For these reasons, the pursuit of patient safety extended towards approaches that promote involvement of front line clinicians in designing 'bottom-up' service solutions.

Thus, the late 1990s saw the advent of two new initiatives. One was clinical pathways, introduced to health care in the early to mid-1990s (Pearson et al. 1995). Formulated by front line clinicians themselves, pathways are descriptions of local clinical practices that formalize and systematize the processes, the sequence and the components of care and associated resource utilization (Campbell et al. 1998). Pathways have served to systematize care in areas such as vascular surgery, hip and knee arthroplasty (Archer et al. 1997, Becker et al. 1997, Dowsey et al. 1999), with fractured neck of femur treatment providing the most prominent example of pathway use (Gallagher 1994). Pathways have produced demonstrated gains in efficiency, effectiveness and efficacy (Archer et al. 1997). They are of special utility in the coordination of multidisciplinary teams. By coordinating different professionals' activities, pathways have shown to reduce errors of omission, length of stay and mortality and morbidity that can be produced by delays.

Pathways also play an important role in gathering information about treatment variations or outliers. This makes pathway design an important pillar of quality and safety improvement (Pinder et al. 2005). This aspect leads into a second initiative, introduced later in the 1990s, under the aegis of 'continuous (quality) improvement' (CQI). CQI was borrowed, like pathways, from industries other than health care. CQI centres on front line staff evaluating selected aspects of their practice and devising interventions to resolve key problems. Pathways allow identification of quality and safety problems because they render outlier practices visible. Complementing this approach, CQI brings front line clinicians together in investigation teams or improvement collaboratives (Bagian et al. 2002), to target specific outlier problems. The pathway approach is holistic in orientation: it seeks to account for the totality of a clinical treatment. In contrast, problem-focused improvement methods are selective (in terms of the problems or failures targeted for improvement).

The approaches to patient safety discussed thus far have the following in common: they are oriented to simplifying the work into ideal principles: guidelines, protocols, pathways or improvement trajectories. This is done on the assumption that humans can and will make errors and that simplification obviates errors. This approach strikes me as self-evident. For decades, automation and mechanization have been the mainstays of how industries and institutions have organized the production of goods and services. Product and service quality and safety are a function of process standardization. For these reasons, health care quality and safety experts and policy-makers have looked to commercial industries and services for answers to how to deal with the rising complexity of care organizations. How else to handle the growing numbers of patients with multiple co-morbidities, requiring access to more and more coordinated forms of treatment supported by more powerful (and therefore often quite dangerous) technologies? How else to manage the services that these patients enter into and which have rising levels of staff turnover and resource allocation and budgeting pressures? To cope with these challenges and 'tame' their complexity (Woods et al. 2007), it seems natural to seek to streamline their care processes, minimize 'waste' (Lean Enterprise Academy UK 2006), and reconcile clinical practices with guidelines, protocols through imposing forcing functions (Norman 1988).

However, recent studies have pointed to 'the implementation gap' and 'undershoot' affecting existing evidence-based guidelines and practice improvement initiatives (Bevan et al. 2007). Delivery of care still corresponds in only around 50 per cent of cases to guidelines and standards (McGlynn et al. 2003, Shojania and Grimshaw 2005). Commentators have pointed to the resistance of professional-clinical subcultures to realise reform: their 'subcultural' divergences obviate effective communication (Degeling et al. 2003). Others have raised the issue of a lack of resources to fund the extra work that is to be done by clinicians to respond to the various patient safety demands: they are simply too busy to change the ways they work (Lemieux-Charles and Hall 1997). Recently, however, different questions have been raised about the approaches described above and about the solutions they offer.

These questions target the very basis of the approaches discussed thus far: the notion that simplifying, planning and statistically measuring work processes are the principal guarantors for service safety and quality. Humans can and will err, of course, and well-executed plans and routines can be a source of safety and quality. But compliance with routines and plans does not necessarily rule out failure and error. Neither do work-arounds (Gasser 1986), or occasions of non-compliance with routines and plans, spell failure. On the contrary, *in situ* creativity and flexibility are often needed to handle multiple challenges happening at the same time. This is recognized in scholarship that provides instances of resilience (Wears et al. 2008), 'error wisdom' (Reason 2004) and 'mindfulness' (Weick 2004).

These latter notions point to the work clinicians need to enact to bridge the gap between *in situ* work and the formal resources with which or through which they are to structure their work (Strauss et al. 1963). Scholarship that analyses this gap demonstrates that routines and plans that are generally hailed as solutions to problems are per definition insensitive to complexities that emerge *in situ*. They require 'articulation' to situations where staff need to 'think on their feet' (Iedema et al. 2006a). Therefore, while important for structuring staff practices and limiting practice variation (Lillrank and Liukko 2004), pre-designed health care processes are in and for themselves no guarantor for *in situ* patient safety (West 2000, Bosk et al. 2009).

Commentators who have begun to acknowledge that the efficacy of routines and plans is contingent on teams' *in situ* adaptability also now begin to revisit our assumptions about the methods and approaches that produce these routines and plans. In an article that reassesses the role of formal scientific investigation in reducing the risks affecting patients, Berwick recently promoted ordinary social knowledge and everyday interpersonal relationships as critical to enabling clinicians to negotiate complexity *in situ*:

> Broadly framed, much of human learning relies wisely on effective approaches to problem solving, learning, growth and development that are different from the types of formal science so well explicated and defended by the scions of evidence-based medicine. Although they are far from RCTs in design, some of those approaches offer good defences against misinterpretation, bias, and confounding. In the world of clinical care, especially in the quest for improvement of clinical processes, is it plausible that those approaches – the ones we use in everyday life – might have value too, used well and consciously, to help us learn? The answer is yes. And yet, the very success of the movement towards formal scientific methods that has matured into the modern commitment to evidence-based medicine now creates a wall that excludes too much of the knowledge and practice that can be harvested from experience itself, reflected upon.

> Berwick (2005: 315–316)

Berwick goes on to list 'using local knowledge', 'integrating detailed process knowledge', 'inviting observers to comment on what they notice rather than "blinding" them against what they know', and 'using small samples' as principles for engaging with questions of patient safety. It is here that an expansion becomes apparent from the paradigm that focuses on anchoring safety to routines, rules and plans, and a new paradigm that regards the full complexity of care practices as needing complementary resources, such as resilience, error wisdom, mindfulness and reflexivity. In the next section of this chapter I present approaches that render visible and thereby promote these latter capabilities. As will become clear, these approaches pay heed to Berwick's emphasis on taking people's local knowledge seriously, and involving lay observers in accomplishing patient safety, including patients and families.

A Complementary Paradigm

This section of this chapter turns to an exploration of a paradigm that targets 'knowledge for theory and practice' (Van De Ven and Johnson 2006); that is, practice-change knowledge that straddles formal routines and plans and *in situ* complexity. This paradigm embodies slightly different approaches, each of which lays claim to noteworthy – if apparently 'merely local' – achievements.[1] Collectively, these approaches complement the ones described in the previous section. Thus, they foreground rather than background what is specific about those who provide care, where it is provided, to whom and with what clinical outcomes and experiential effects. Likewise, they respect and privilege multiple stakeholders' perspectives. By respecting the views and experiences of clinicians, patients, relatives, managers and so forth, debates over principles and quests for consensus are transformed into shared dialogues that afford flexibility, variation, and compromise.

Three approaches are discussed: (1) organizational redesign, (2) expansive learning and (3) video-reflexive ethnography. The first, organizational redesign, derives from the science of designing technologies and environments. The main principles of organizational redesign are analysis and prototyping (Coughlan et al. 2007). In organizational redesign, analysis moves beyond methods that distance the researcher from the people and the practices that are being studied (such as surveys and questionnaires). Analysis, here, centres on involving researchers and practitioners in reflecting on stories told and depictions produced about the work (Boyle and Pratt 2004).

These stories and depictions serve an important purpose besides representing current work processes: they prototype alternative ways of working. Prototyping

---

1   *In situ* practice change as conceptualized here rarely remains 'merely local' because of the entanglement among actors that it affords and inspires. See the Discussion section for more elaboration.

involves constructing alternative models for future practice through feedback and trialling. These models have an experimental function; they enable the practitioner to act out new ways of working, during which learning results from 'being given the opportunity to explore new behaviours and new ideas and activities [that are allowed to fail] "faster, early and often"' (Coughlan et al. 2007: 127). Service redesign, then, is not achieved instantly but involves ongoing experimentation. In organizational redesign, the monitoring of how redesigned models impact on practices relies on 'self-reflection, action research and narrative interventions' (Trullen and Bartunek 2007: 33).

In a recent book on the subject, Bate and Robert (2007) use the labels 'organizational redesign' and 'experience-based design' interchangeably, linking organizational and individual foci in an ongoing dialogue focused on designing common ground. Their approach involves the patient and the practitioner ('user') in collectively remodelling clinical practices. This cooperation is informed by the knowledge that design harbours three values: functionality (performance), reliability (engineering) and aesthetics (experience). Bate and Robert emphasize that organizational redesign aims to keep the technologically oriented aims of functionality and reliability in balance with that of aesthetics, or of patients' experience of and responses to the new design:

> In its own way, health care has always been quite deeply involved with the first two elements of design: 'performance' in terms of the use of evidence-based practice, pathways and process design to ensure the clinical intervention is right; and 'engineering' in terms of clinical governance and standards to make it safer and more reliable (although making it *feel* safe may be a different matter) ... But arguably health care has never engaged explicitly or anything like the same extent with the third element – designing human experiences (as distinct from designing processes).
>
> Bate and Robert (2007: 17)

Bate and Robert's concern with patients' personal experiences is what distinguishes organizational design from approaches that privilege clinical, organizational, scientific and technological factors, such as work domain mapping and task analysis (Vicente 2000). By introducing patient experiences as a design factor, Bate and Robert render legitimate personal and affective responses to new practice prototypes.

By way of example, let us consider the following description of a moment when 'both patient and staff member identify and corroborate a touch point where improvements to patient experience could and need to be made' (Bate and Robert 2007: 151). The 'touch point' discussed between the patient and the oncologist is the breaking of bad news:

Patient: Everybody does things their own way, but I would have done it differently.

Oncologist: The diagnosis, the treatment options discussion, those are very defining moments so I think we could organize the clinic better so that we don't have three or four people being told bad news and having treatment options all discussed at the same time ... I think we need to train everybody to break it a bit better. I don't think I am in any way perfect at doing it, I know I'm not very good at doing it, but at least I've had some training on how to do it.

Bate and Robert (2007: 151)

Bate and Robert's comment on these statements is that 'in this case, both patient and oncologist clearly agreed that this is one touch point that needs to be addressed in the department's experience design process' (Bate and Robert 2007: 151). Though their work is still ongoing, they point out that:

Many of the individual co-design groups have continued to 'recruit' new patients and carers thereby broadening the experiences upon which the group can draw to identify and improve touch points. Many seemingly minor changes (for example, moving the weighing scales), which were found to be impacting in a significant way on patient experiences, were actioned almost immediately; other issues (for example, levels of staff training on the post-operative ward) are being addressed through longer-term solutions. Members of the core team meet regularly with the chief executive of the hospital to (a) ensure that the ongoing work is integrated into the wider improvement efforts of the organization, and (b) anchor the identified priorities into the performance management systems in the hospital.

Bate and Robert (2007: 156)

Experience-based design has since expanded into 'co-design', an approach that brings practitioners and patients together to redesign process or facility aspects of care. Co-design does not limit itself to improving patients' experiences and the quality of care. It also seeks solutions that enhance patients' safety (Iedema et al. 2010a). Co-design, in turn, thanks to its emphasis on bringing different stakeholders together in new 'forums of engagement' (Latour 2004), is a close relative of Engeström's (1999) expansive learning, to which I turn now.

Developed by Engeström and colleagues at the University of Helsinki, expansive learning is characterized by four distinct phases (Engeström 1999). Learning begins with highlighting disturbances and contradictions that are embedded in work practices. These disturbances and contradictions are made visible through collecting (visual) data about how patients and practitioners speak and act, and analysing the footage. Then, researchers, patients and practitioners come together to explore the implications that follow from these data analyses and articulate alternative work activities. The third phase centres on designing, experimenting and implementing new practices, and phase four focuses on revisiting the intended and unintended consequences of decisions taken. As does Bate and Robert's work, Engeström and colleagues' work takes *in situ* problems as its point of departure, and creates sites where researchers and researchees can come together to engage with specific problems and explore new opportunities.

The model of expansive learning was applied in one project to the consultation processes that occurred in General Practitioners' (GPs) clinics. Engeström used video data to engender practitioners' insight into and reflection on existing processes (Engeström 2003). In more recent work, Engeström and his team proactively arranged encounters among GP's, patients and acute care specialists, with the aim of improving continuity of care for geriatric patients. They used video data to capture obstacles in the care continuum (Engeström et al. 2003, Kerosuo 2007), as well as using video data as feedback to elicit practitioners' and patients' views and reflections about their work.

One specific and noteworthy achievement, first discussed in their 2003 publication (Engeström et al. 2003), is the shared design of a 'care calendar'. The care calendar arose from discussions among the GP, the specialist and the patient following their reflections on footage of their ways of working and communicating. The footage made new conversations possible among these stakeholders, revisiting and redesigning the routines defining their care communication processes (Kerosuo 2007). The care calendar became a critical mediating instrument, straddling, connecting and reinventing stakeholders' communication and perspectives. The communication elicited through reflection translated into a shared creation of care continuity, with the care calendar acting as symbol of stakeholders' newfound relationship, agreement and plan.

The learning principle at work in Engeström's studies derives from researchers, practitioners and patients considering research data together. They all thereby gain the opportunity to reflect on the logic of existing practices. Because the footage shows them in action, their reflections tie straight into their personal lives and identities, enabling conduct change. This reflexive process tests the accuracy and comprehensiveness of their understandings and conclusions, and enables them to conceptualize innovative solutions as well as experiment in practice with alternatives – hence, 'expansive learning'.

Expansive learning through feedback and reflexive engagement is also prominent in the third approach showcased here: video-reflexive ethnography. What distinguishes this method from the first two is that before doing anything else, it foregrounds the creation of social relationships – 'entanglement' – among researchers and 'researchees'. Video-reflexive ethnography is contingent on entanglement as the principal condition for researchers and practitioners to develop shared attentiveness to particular problems and struggles, insight into alternatives and engagement with and commitment to change initiatives. Entanglement comes about as a result of investing time with practitioners at work, and with patients as they move through care. In that regard, this third approach to learning delves into both the details of existing practices and into the complexities and dynamics of relationships (Iedema et al. 2006b, 2006c, 2009a).

Examples of achievements here include clinicians' engagement with infection-control risks (Iedema and Rhodes 2010), their improvement in handover practice (Carroll et al. 2008, Iedema et al. 2009b), enhanced attention to complex care issues (Iedema et al. 2006d) and restructured communicative relationships away from medical dominance and more in line with 'clinical democracy' (Long et al. 2006). To flesh out one of these examples, let us consider the infection control study in greater detail. In the extract below, an Infection Control Clinical Nurse Consultant is speaking to local metropolitan teaching hospital staff about the benefits of video-ethnographic intervention:

> In 2003 our MRSA rate that they acquired within the acute spinal unit was ... 38 acquisitions for 2003 ... In 2005, I was actually doing a lot of work within the spinal unit and I started the project, it went down to 27 and I can tell you up to the end of Sep ... well today, up to today, 2006, we've gone down to 7 MRSA. So that I think alone tells you, the implications that this had. And you might think well, why has this study had a huge implication and I'll tell you why. It's because they've taken ownership of multi ... of acquisition of infections within that unit. It's no longer my issue, it's their issue. And this is what this project's helped them to do.

Infection Control Nurse 22 October 2006

The video-reflexive ethnographic study that elicited this remark unfolded as follows. When attending a video-reflexive session during which staff were shown footage of their own ward practices, the nurse speaking above realized that the visual data harboured valuable information that she was unable to access otherwise. When practising infection-control surveillance on the ward by observing 'live' caring practices, the nurse was unable to see what she saw in the footage displayed on the screen.

Research into how practitioners and patients respond to footage suggests that viewing such film has a transformative impact on their experience and enactment of social processes, relationships and identities (Massumi 2002, MacDougall 2006). This transformative impact derives from clinicians seeing themselves in the footage as 'third persons', or as others seen by themselves. This perspective objectifies what for them has always remained within the bounds of taken-as-given experience. At the same time, the experience of seeing oneself as another sees one also intensifies the viewing experience. People frequently express surprise and disbelief at what they see, even if they have 'lived' the situations they are viewing for years. Moreover, they generally feel enabled to act on their own practices and change the ways they work and act. In sum, video enables them to see why change is needed and where. In that way, this method entrusts them with the responsibility for redesigning their work (Carroll et al. 2008, Iedema et al. 2009b).

The results of the infection-control study were dramatic (Iedema and Rhodes 2010). One intriguing learning point here is that infection control may be contingent in a significant way not just on hand-washing, but on how clinicians communicate with one another – if not linguistically, then at least through how they enact their bodily relationships, how they handle medical and communicative–informational technologies (records, letters, phones) and other resources (gloves, gowns, bed handrails), and how they conduct themselves with respect to potentially infectious wounds and patients. More importantly still, participants' attentiveness appeared enhanced through shared narration of experiences in response to visual accounts of *in situ* practices and processes. It is the social relations that result, or the weave of affect that these video-feedback sessions engendered, rather than purely formal knowing and remembering, that is at the heart of video-reflexive ethnography, and central to this unit's ability to augment its outcomes (Iedema et al. 2006c).

Discussion – Implications

> Perception is exactly proportioned to its action upon the thing.

> Massumi (2002: 90)

The approaches just discussed differ paradigmatically from the bureaucratic, scientific and collaborative ones described earlier in this chapter. The latter were characterized as centring on the roll-out of set solutions, best practice evidence and rules devised from the new knowledge obtained. Such formal knowledge provides direction and guidance for staff, providing information they can and should fall back on. But compliance with such knowledge and rules does not guarantee safe care. It is here that this first patient safety paradigm runs up against an inbuilt limit.

Indeed, this paradigm produces two separate but related challenges. First, it projects order and stasis onto a field of practice that is dynamic to the point of frequently being experienced as lacking order and structure. Front line staff make proximate choices all the time about how a rule or a fact applies in practice. They inevitably confront the problem that having a rule or fact does not equate with knowing how to apply it: '[t]he ability to reduce everything to simple fundamental laws does not imply [that people have] the ability to start from those laws and reconstruct the universe' (Woods 2007: 47). Second, thanks to its concern with formalized knowledge and rules, this first paradigm risks downplaying what front line clinicians do to make those rules and facts relevant to the here and now. This paradigm also backgrounds what they do over and above knowledge application and rule compliance. That is, the creative flexibility they need to muster and display to overcome complex challenges and avoid impending risks. The existing patient safety policy and research agenda allows this first paradigm to prevail, and regards problems arising *in situ* as to do with organizational leadership, team culture or personal character.

What is needed is a complementary perspective. This perspective does not just recognize that individuals make their own specific, local decisions, thereby activating specific rules and ignoring others. It also recognizes that individuals are integral to rule-making; the insights and wisdom they derive from doing their work come to structure the rules that govern that work (Iedema 2003). Here, what practitioners do and the rules they apply are not entirely separate domains. This transpires when practitioners reflect on and discuss how they enact relationships and processes that involve professionals and patients and carers. Through reflecting on these relationships and processes, they become aware of the links (and gaps) between micro-clinical processes and large-scale organizational trajectories; between local ways of working and overarching rules and systems. When acting in alignment with this second paradigm, practitioners have come to terms with what they as professionals were taught not (or no longer) to see: the mundane, everyday ways in which relationships and processes are acted out, what that means for them and for their patients and what implications these local ways of acting have for overarching organizational rules.

This second paradigm does not regard simplification and generalization as focal principles. It positions rules and facts as constantly in tension with local complexity and the dynamics of *in situ* processes. At the same time, this second paradigm explores how to teach practitioners to recognize and engage with dynamic complexity – that is, becoming more sensitized or heedful to the contexts, processes and individuals that confront them (Weick and Roberts 1993). In essence, this paradigm does not privilege the production of new abstract knowledge per se, but foregrounds the importance of focusing on how practitioners negotiate such knowledge and rules with others in local contexts. For this to happen, what is needed is people's attention to and sharing of how they and those around them understand, deploy and adapt such knowledge and rules.

Here, the discussion connects with the question of method. The second paradigm favours narrative, visual and participatory methods. These are not specifically research or improvement methods – they do both (research and improvement). The critical principle is that viewing themselves and narrating their experiences to and with each other, people come to embody a new structure of attention (Thrift 2004a). This new structure of attention is both the medium and the outcome of fellow clinicians and patients sharing experiences and perspectives, rendering these newly visible and tangible, and being prepared to consider these relevant enough for inclusion into new organizational rules.

This brings me to a final, methodological point. The first paradigm lends itself to 'spread' because of its preoccupation with producing reliable and portable knowledge from rigourous and replicable methods. However, the 'rigour' that underpins this paradigm and its methods sets up an a priori distance between researchers and researched, and between the improvers and what needs to be improved. If viewed through the lens of Massumi's quotation above – the way we perceive something determines how and whether we can act on it – we realize the decision to impose rigour has advantages as well as disadvantages. To be sure, distance from what we seek to improve and act on is important for creating portable knowledge and rules, but it also extricates this knowledge and these rules from everyday experience and emotional engagement. And that is the inevitable disadvantage inherent in rigourous research. This disadvantage becomes an acute problem in situations of high and rising complexity. There, people are increasingly called on to find solutions for new or 'emergent' problems. In complex contexts, then, formal knowledge and rules need to be accompanied with other and increasingly important skills: interpersonal attentiveness, flexible responsiveness and skilful and effective communication.

Given that it engages with practitioners, patients and other stakeholders at the level of local complexity, the second paradigm outlined here may be able to make a special claim about its ability to facilitate and encourage general spread. Here, knowledge travels through mundane experience shared through stories, or the kind of everyday communication and sensibility that Berwick (2005) and others have now begun to promote as central to patient safety. This rising interest in stories and narrative[2] is not surprising. Narrative harnesses the force, economy and immediacy of interpersonal affect that is shared constantly by actors in everyday life. Indeed, affect is the principal basis and medium of human sociality (Massumi 2002), because in contrast to the channels open to formal knowledge, 'affect is ... a very time-efficient way of transmitting a large amount of information' (Thrift 2004b: 878).

Foregrounding affect, the second paradigm engages with the experiential dimension of being, with how people relate and (inter)act. It highlights the importance of contextualized, informal and dynamic (changeable) kinds of knowing and planning. It confronts the messiness and changeability of *in situ* activity: the contestations, disagreements, uncertainties and tensions. It highlights the importance of friendships, bonds and loyalties, but also of a new structure of attention that is increasingly needed in contemporary kinds of work as people straddle multiple professional, social and cultural boundaries.

All this represents an important shift in thinking about patient safety towards relations and affect. We take seriously the role of affect as both means and condition of communication (Iedema et al 2009c). In acknowledging the importance of affect, it is recognized that good patient care is contingent not just on accurate information and formal guidance, but also on the experiential dimensions of practice and safety: social relationships (Bate 2004), care (Mol 2008), civility (Woods 2007), heedfulness and mindfulness (Weick 2004) – all modes of social, practical and interpersonal entanglement (Iedema and Carroll 2010).

What does this mean for practice? Approaches belonging to the second paradigm can be integrated with clinical practice in different ways. First, experiential and

---

2   Distinction can be drawn between the terms story and narrative (Herman 2004), but I will treat these terms as synonymous for now.

narrative kinds of enquiry can enrich clinical service redesign initiatives (Iedema et al. 2010a). Both experience-based enquiry and expansive learning already offer powerful examples of retrospective and proactive service reforms. Second, as video-reflexive ethnography has begun to show, clinicians and patients themselves become interested in research skill transfer, with video methodologies being adopted and integrated in the teaching and learning approaches used by infection control staff (Long et al. 2006), the enhancement of clinical handover (Iedema et al. 2009c) and the promotion of incident disclosure (Iedema et al. 2010b). This also points to the importance of people moving across community, clinical, policy and academic boundaries (Iedema and Carroll 2011). These movements can take the form of patients collaborating with academics on developing new perspectives on care trajectories, clinicians taking time out to work in-house with researchers on work-specific problems, or of practitioners taking up temporary positions or 'externships' working alongside health services researchers on more general issues. Now that workplace learning has been recognized to be most effective if it ties in with people's experiential and narrative realities (Boud and Miller 1996), it seems natural to capitalize on those methods and approaches that delve into the actual life worlds of clinicians and patients.

Conclusion

Many arguments have been mobilized in favour of the paradigm that targets the production of evidence, knowledge and rules. These arguments have centred on needing to target the prevailing patient safety risks and predominant preventable incidents, such as falls, medication errors and hospital-acquired infections. Knowledge of these risks enables us to devise systems that minimize incidents associated with those risks (Runciman et al 2001). We now also know that safe practice is not purely a function of constraining and regulating individuals' access to formal knowledge, ensuring they follow ritualized procedures, or respect predesigned forcing functions. Truly safe ways of working are also contingent on people's interpersonal sensitivities and social responsiveness (Gherardi and Nicolini 2002). Commentators in the area of organizational safety research now talk about these sensitivities and responsiveness using terms like 'resilience' (Hollnagel et al. 2006), 'heedfulness' (Weick and Roberts 1993), and 'error wisdom' (Reason 2004). Collectively, these notions underscore the significance for safe practice of relational or affect-based conducts (Thrift 2004a).

Affect-based conducts underpin the possibility of individuals being open to noticing problems and tensions in the 'here-and-now', and acting on these. As recent work on hospital corridor spaces has shown, the affective nature of clinicians' relationships plays a crucial role in whether they are able to register and engage with processual obstacles and gaps (Iedema et al. 2010c). Whether manifesting as respect, resilience, mindfulness, care or compassion, affect is a precondition for learning. This is a crucial point, given informal conditions and exchanges are now recognized to be the most economic and effective sites of workplace learning (Boud and Miller 1996). The patient safety literature is now beginning to engage with these matters, leading to more sophisticated discussions about the role of prescriptions and proscriptions for practice (Bosk et al. 2009, Mesman 2008a, 2008b, 2009).

The patient safety literature now recognizes the importance of affect-based conducts in its concern with culture, leadership, teamwork and trust – the quadrivium of quality of care and patient safety. It is exciting to see that discussions about these matters begin to drill down into how people act and communicate *in situ*, acknowledging that what happens there has important consequences for the overall system, care experience, quality and safety. This calls for new partnerships between practitioners, patients, researchers and policy-makers – partnerships that break down boundaries between knowledge generation and practice improvement, and between experience-based co-design and systems design. Indeed, if the experiential and affect-based dimensions of social practice and human relationships are crucial to realizing patient safety (Gherardi and Nicolini 2002), should we not also re-think the methods we draw on to understand and enhance patients' safety?

Acknowledgements

This research has been made possible thanks to three Discovery grants from the Australian Research Council (DP0450773, DP0556438 and DP0879002) led by Rick Iedema.

References

Archer, S.B., Burnett, R.J., Flesch, L.V., Hobler, S.C., Bower, R.H., Nussbaum, M.S. and Fischer, J.E. 1997. Implementation of a clinical pathway decreases length of stay and hospital charges for patients undergoing total colectomy and ileal pounch/anal anastomosis. *Surgery*, 122(4), 699–703, Discussion pp. 703–705.

Bagian, J.P., Gosbee, J., Lee, C.Z., Williams, L., McKnight, S.D. and Mannos, D.M. 2002. The Veterans Affairs Root Cause Analysis system in action. *Journal on Quality Improvement*, 28, 531–545.

Bate, P. 2004. The role of stories and storytelling in organizational change efforts: the anthropology of an intervention within a UK hospital. *Intervention Research*, 1(2004), 27–42.

Bate, P. and Robert, G. 2007. *Bringing User Experience to Healthcare Improvement: The Concepts, Methods And Practices Of Experience-Based Design.* Oxford/ Seattle: Radcliffe Publishing.

Becker, B.N., Breiterman-White, R., Van Buren, D. Fotiadis, C., Richie, R.E. and Schulman, G. 1997. Care pathway reduces hospitalisations and cost for haemodialysis vascular access surgery. *American Journal of Kidney Disease*, 30(4), 525–531.

Berwick, D. 1998. Beyond survival: towards continuous improvement in medical care. *New Horizons*, 6(1), 3–11.

Berwick, D. 2005. Broadening the view of evidence-based medicine. *Quality and Safety in Health Care*, 14(5), 315–316.

Bevan, H., Bate, P. and Robert, G. 2007. Using a design approach to assist large-scale organizational change. *Journal of Applied Behavioral Science*, 43(1), 135–152.

Bosk, C.L., Dixon-Woods, M., Goeschel, C. and Pronovost, P. 2009. The art of medicine: reality check for checklists. *Lancet*, 374, 444–445.

Boud, D. and Miller, N. 1996. *Working with Experience: Animating Learning*. London: Routledge.

Boyle, S. and Pratt, J. 2004. Agent-based working: a device for systemic dialogue. In: *Complexity and Health Care Organisation: A View from the Street*, edited by D. Kernick. Oxford: Radcliffe Medical Press, pp. 159–170.

Campbell, H., Hotchkiss, R., Bradshaw, N. and Porteous, M. 1998. Integrated care pathways. *British Medical Journal*, 316, 133–137.

Carroll, K., Iedema, R. and Kerridge, R. 2008. Reshaping ICU ward round practices using video reflexive ethnography. *Qualitative Health Research*, 18(3), 380–390.

Cook, R.I. and Woods, D.D. 1994. Operating at the sharp end: the complexity of human error. In: *Human Error in Medicine*, edited by S. Bogner. Mahwah: Lawrence Erlbaum, pp. 255–310.

Coughlan, P., Fulton-Suri, J. and Canales, K. 2007. Prototypes as (design) tools for behavioral and organizational change. *Journal of Applied Behavioral Science*, 43(1), 122–134.

Degeling, P., Maxwell, S., Kennedy, J. and Coyle, B. 2003. Medicine, management and modernisation: a 'danse macabre'? *British Medical Journal*, 326, 649–652.

Department of Health. 2000. *An Organisation With A Memory: Report of an Expert Group on Learning from Adverse Events in The NHS, Chaired by the Chief Medical Officer*. London: The Stationery Office.

Dowsey, M., Kilgour, M., Sanatamaria, N. and Choong, P. 1999. Clinical pathways in hip and knee arthrosplasty: a prospective randomised controlled study. *Medical Journal of Australia*, 170(2), 59–62.

Engeström, Y. 1999. Expansive visibilization of work: an activity-theoretical perspective. *The Journal of Collaborative Computing*, 8(1), 63–93.

Engeström, Y., Engeström, R. and Kerosuo, H. 2003. The discursive construction of collaborative care. *Applied Linguistics*, 24(3), 286–315.

Gallagher, C. 1994. Applying quality improvement tools to quality planning: paediatric femur fracture clinical path development. *Journal for Healthcare Quality*, 16(3), 6–14.

Gasser, L. 1986. The integration of computing and routine work. *ACM Transactions on Office Information Systems*, 4, 205–225.

Gherardi, S. and Nicolini, D. (2002). Learning the trade: a culture of safety in practice. *Organization*, 9(2), 191–223.

Herman, D. 2004. *Story Logic: Problems And Possibilities Of Narrative*. Lincoln: University of Nebraska Press.

Hollnagel, E., Woods, D.D. and Leveson, N. 2006. *Resilience Engineering: Concepts And Precepts*. Aldershot: Ashgate Publishing Ltd.

Iedema, R. (2011). Creating safety by strengthening clinicians' capacity for reflexivity. *BMJ Quality and Safety*, 20(Suppl 1), i83–i86.

Iedema, R. 2003. *Discourses of Post-Bureaucratic Organization*. Amsterdam/ Philadelphia: John Benjamins.

Iedema, R. and Carroll, K. (2011). The 'clinalyst': institutionalizing reflexive space to realize safety and flexible systematization in health care. *Journal of Organizational Change Management*, 24(2), 175–190.

Iedema, R. and Carroll, K. 2010. Discourse research that intervenes in the quality and safety of clinical practice. *Discourse & Communication*, 4(1), 68–86.

Iedema, R. and Rhodes, C. (2010). An ethics of mutual care in organizational surveillance. *Organization Studies*, 31(2), 199–217.

Iedema, R., Allen, S., Britton, K., Gallagher, T., Piper, D., Sloan, T., et al. 2010b. *Final Report: The '100 Patient Stories' Project including Indicators of Effective Open Disclosure and Open Disclosure Fundamentals*. Sydney: UTS Centre for Health Communication and Australian Commission for Safety and Quality in Health Care.

Iedema, R., Forsyth, R., Georgiou, A., Braithwaite, J. and Westbrook, J. 2006b. Video research in health: visibilizing the normative and affective complexities of contemporary care. *Qualitative Research Journal*, 6(2), 15–30.

Iedema, R., Jorm, C. and Lum, M. 2009c. Affect is central to patient safety: the horror stories of young anaesthetists. *Social Science & Medicine*, 69(12), 1750–1756.

Iedema, R., Jorm, C.M., Braithwaite, J., Travaglia, J. and Lum, M. 2006a. A root cause analysis of clinical errors: confronting the disjunction between formal rules and situated clinical activity. *Social Science & Medicine*, 63(5), 1201–1212.

Iedema, R., Long, D. and Carroll, K. 2010c. Corridor communication, spatial design and patient safety: enacting and managing complexities. In: *Space, Meaning and Organisation*, edited by A. van Marrewijk and D. Yanow. Cheltenham: Edward Elgar, pp. 41–57.

Iedema, R., Long, D., Carroll, K., Stenglin, M. and Braithwaite, J. 2006d. *Corridor Work: How Liminal Space Becomes a Resource for Handling Complexity in Healthcare*. Paper presented at the Australian-Pacific Researchers in Organization Studies Conference.

Iedema, R., Long, D., Forsyth, R. and Lee, B. 2006c. Visibilizing clinical work: video ethnography in the contemporary hospital. *Health Sociology Review*, 15(2), 156–168.

Iedema, R., Merrick, E., Kerridge, R., Herkes, R., Lee, B., Anscombe, M., et al. 2009b. 'Handover – Enabling Learning in Communication for Safety' (HELiCS): a report on achievements at two hospital sites. *Medical Journal of Australia*, 190(11), S133–S136.

Iedema, R., Merrick, E., Piper, D., Britton, K., Gray, J., Verma, R., et al. 2010a. Co-design as discursive practice in emergency health services: the architecture of deliberation. *Journal of Applied Behavioural Science*, 46, 73–91.

Iedema, R., Merrick, E., Rajbhandari, D., Gardo, A., Stirling, A. and Herkes, R. 2009a. Viewing the taken-for-granted from under a different aspect: a video-based method in pursuit of patient safety. *International Journal for Multiple Research Approaches*, 3(3), 290–301.

Institute of Medicine. 2001. *Crossing The Quality Chasm: A New Health System For The 21st Century*. Washington: National Academy Press.

Kerosuo, H. 2007. Renegotiating disjunctions in inter-organizationally provided care. In: *The Discourse of Hospital Communication: Tracing Complexities in Contemporary Health Care Organizations*, edited by R. Iedema. Basingstoke: Palgrave-Macmillan, pp. 138–161.

Latour, B. 2004. Why has critique run out of steam? From matters of fact to matters of concern. *Critical Enquiry*, 30, 225–248.

Lean Enterprise Academy UK. 2006. *Lean Thinking for the NHS*. Coventry: NHS Institute of Innovation and Improvement.

Leatherman, S. 2007. *Health System Reform: Using Evidence for Improving Quality and Performance*. Paper presented at the National Institute of Clinical Studies.

Lemieux-Charles, L. and Hall, M. 1997. When resources are scarce: the impact of three organisational practices on clinician-managers. *Health Care Management Review*, 22(1), 58–69.

Lillrank, P. and Liukko, M. 2004. Standard, routine and non-routine processes in health care. *International Journal of Health Care Quality Assurance*, 17(1), 39–46.

Lomas, J., Enkin, M., Anderson, G., Hannah, W.J., Vayda, E. and Singer, J. 1991. Opinion leaders vs audit and feedback to implement practice guidelines. *Journal of the American Medical Association*, 265(17), 2202–2207.

Long, D., Clezy, K., Pontovivo, G., Lee, B. and Iedema, R. 2006. *Preventing Health Care Associated Infections: A Novel Approach Using Ethnography*. Paper presented at the Australasian Society for Infectious Diseases Conference, Wellington New Zealand.

Long, D., Forsyth, R., Carroll, K. and Iedema, R. (2006). The (im)possibility of clinical democracy. *Health Sociology Review*, 15(5), 506–519.

MacDougall, D. 2006. *The Corporeal Image: Film, Ethnography And The Senses*. Princeton: Princeton University Press.

Massumi, B. 2002. *Parables For The Virtual: Movement, Affect, Sensation.* Durham: Duke University Press.

McGlynn, E.A., Asch, S.M., Adams, J., Keesey, J., Hicks, J., DeCristofaro, A., et al. 2003. The quality of health care delivered to adults in the United States. *New England Journal of Medicine*, 348(26), 2635–2645.

McLaughlin, J. 2001. EBM and risk: rhetorical resources in the articulation of professional identity. *Journal of Management in Medicine*, 15(5), 352–363.

Meek, J. 2001. Brave new world of life and hope. *Sydney Morning Herald*, 18 October 2001, 15.

Mesman, J. 2008a. *Experienced Pioneers: Uncertainty and Medical Innovation in Neonatology.* Basingstoke: Palgrave-Macmillan.

Mesman, J. 2008b. *Uncertainty in Medical Innovation: Experienced Pioneers in Neonatal Care.* Basingstoke: Palgrave MacMillan.

Mesman, J. 2009. The geography of patient safety: a topical analysis of sterility. *Social Science and Medicine*, 69(12), 705–1712.

Mol, A. 2008. *The Logic of Care.* London: Routledge.

Norman, D.A. 1988. *The Psychology of Everyday Things.* New York: Basic Books.

Pain, C. and Lord, R. 2006. Lessons from Campbelltown and Camden hospitals. *ANZ Journal of Surgery*, 76 (Suppl 1), A42–A44.

Pearson, S., Goulart-Fischer, D. and Lee, T. 1995. Critical pathways as a strategy for improving care: problems and potential. *Annals of Internal Medicine*, 123(12), 941–948.

Pinder, R., Petchey, R., Shaw, S. and Carter, Y. 2005. What's in a care pathway? Towards a cultural cartography of the new NHS. *Sociology of Health and Illness*, 27(6), 759–779.

Reason, J. 2004. Beyond the organizational accident: the need for 'error wisdom' on the frontline. *Journal of Quality and Safety in Health Care*, 13, 28–33.

Runciman, W., Merry, A. and McCall-Smith, A. 2001. Improving patients' safety by gathering information. *British Medical Journal*, 323, 298.

Shojania, K.G. and Grimshaw, J.M. 2005. Evidence-based quality improvement: the state of the science. *Health Affairs*, 24(1), 138–151.

Steinberg, E.P. and Luce, B.R. 2005. Evidence based? Caveat emptor! *Health Affairs*, 24, 80–93.

Strauss, A., Schatzman, L., Ehrlich, D., Bucher, R. and Sabshin, M. 1963. The hospital and its negotiated order. In: *The Hospital in Modern Society*, edited by E. Freidson. New York: Free Press of Glencoe, pp. 147–169.

Tenner, E. 1996. *Why Things Bite Back: Technology and the Revenge Effect.* London: Fourth Estate.

Thrift, N. 2004a. Intensities of feeling: towards a spatial politics of affect. *Geografiska Annaler*, 86B(1), 57–78.

Thrift, N. 2004b. Thick time. *Organization*, 11(6), 873–880.

Trullen, J. and Bartunek, J. 2007. What a design approach offers to organization development. *Journal of Applied Behavioral Science*, 43(1), 23–40.

Van De Ven, A.H. and Johnson, P.E. 2006. Knowledge for theory and practice. *Academy of Management Review*, 31(4), 802–821.

Van Der Weyden, M. 2004. The 'Cam affair': an isolated incident or destined to be repeated? *MJA: Medical Journal of Austalia*, 180(3), 100–101.

Vicente, K.J. 2000. Work domain analysis and task analysis: a difference that matters. In: *Cognitive Task Analysis*, edited by J.M. Schraagen, S.F. Chipman and V.L. Shalin. Mahwah: Erlbaum, pp. 101–118.

Walshe, K. and Boaden, R. (2006). Introduction: patient safety – research into practice. In: *Patient Safety – Research Into Practice*, edited by K. Walshe and R. Boaden. Maidenhead: Open University Press, pp. 1–6.

Wears, R.L., Perry, S.J., Anders, S. and Woods, D. 2008. Resilience in the emergency department. In: *Remaining Sensitive to the Possibility of Failure*, edited by E. Hollnagel, C.P. Nemeth and S.W.A. Dekker. Aldershot: Ashgate, pp. 193–210.

Weick, K. 2004. Reduction of medical errors through mindful interdependence. In: *Medical Error*, edited by K. Sutcliffe and M. Rosenthal. San Francisco: Jossey-Bass, pp. 177–199.

Weick, K. and Roberts, K.H. 1993. Collective mind in organizations: heedful interrelating on flight decks. *Administrative Science Quarterly*, 38, 357–381.

West, E. 2000. Organizational sources of safety and danger: sociological contributions to the study of adverse events. *Quality in Health Care*, 9, 120–126.

Woods, D.D., Patterson, E.S. and Cook, R.I. 2007. Behind human error: taming complexity to improve patient safety. In: *Handbook of Human Factors and Ergonomics in Health Care and Patient Safety*, edited by P. Carayon. Mahwah: Lawrence Erlbaum Associates, pp. 459–476.

Woods, M.S. 2007. *Healing Words: The Power Of Apology In Medicine*. Oakbrook Terrace: Joint Commission on Accreditation of Healthcare Organizations.

Woolf, S.H., Grol, R., Hutchinson, A., Eccles, M. and Grimshaw, J. 1999. Potential benefits, limitations and harms of clinical guidelines. *British Medical Journal*, 318, 527–530.

Concluding Remarks:
The Gaps and Future Directions for Patient Safety Research

Justin Waring and Emma Rowley

On reflection we can see that the field of patient safety research has and continues to mature and evolve. It might be argued that the early years were largely spent trying to highlight the very existence and nature of the problem. Even after the publication of reports such as the Harvard Medical Practice Study (Brennan et al. 1991) the issues of error and safety were often marginal to health services research and policy. The late 1990s witnessed something of a sea change, exemplified by the publication of *To Err is Human* (Institute of Medicine 1999) and then *An Organisation with a Memory* (Department of Health 2000). These reports placed patient safety firmly at the centre of policy-making and service improvement and set in train a decade of sustained research activity and reform. This ranged from conceptual work aimed at changing how we thought about and approached questions of safety (for example Leape 1997, Vincent and Reason 1999, Reason 2000) to strategies, technologies and interventions to enhance safety (for example Waring et al. 2010). Although several authors in this collection are at times critical of the assumptions put forward by this mainstream approach, it is important that we do not forget the essential conceptual, empirical and methodological work undertaken to raise the profile of patient safety, to create a new way of thinking about patient safety, and to stimulate innovations and interventions to improve patient safety.

That being said, the aim of this collection has been to identify and develop areas of patient safety research that have often been neglected by the mainstream. At the outset we interpreted the vast majority of research as being characterized by a 'measure and manage' orthodoxy, which sought to determine the precise nature, frequency and latent sources of risk; to identify the available safety improvements; and then evaluate the application of these solutions. Yet too often this research overlooked or downplayed the social, culture and institutional dimension to patient safety, tending instead towards the more technological or psychological dimensions of safety. Alternatively, where these issues have been addressed they have often been simplified or reified to make them 'fit' with the orthodox approach. For instance, culture remains a central issue to improved patient safety (Lilford 2010), but it is commonly portrayed as a tangible organizational property manifest as espoused attitudes, measured through surveys and as amenable to management intervention. The chapters in this collection address directly what we see as the socio-cultural 'gaps' or missing elements in patient safety research. In doing this they draw on and make connections with a range of social sciences theories and debates that, to date, have had relatively limited exposure in the patient safety community. The themes that organize this collection provide a clear indication of where these gaps exist and where future research might be positioned, including public and patient perspectives, clinical practice, technology, knowledge sharing and learning.

In the theme of public and patient perspectives, Palmer and Murcott's chapter explores the complex, and often paradoxical relationship between the media and patient safety. They show that while the media is active in communicating information in the wake of safety events, sometimes fermenting moral panic, it often pays little attention to the advances and improvements in safety. More broadly their chapter highlights how public and political concern with patient safety is often fuelled by the media. However, Ocloo's chapter questions the extent to which the public and more specifically patients are engaged in the patient safety movement. Drawing parallels with other health and social care movements, she calls for greater recognition of and engagement with groups and agencies that represent and articulate the 'voice' of patients in the advancement of patient safety. Together these chapters reveal to us the way multiple, sometimes competing voices and stakeholder groups are integral to how patient safety emerges as a social issue, but also how these issues can become dominated by particular groups or assumptions to the exclusion of others.

In the theme of clinical practice, Drach-Zahavy and Somech look at nursing policy and practice, arguing that the gap between safety, as determined in policies and guidelines, and on the ground practice, is systemic and predictable. They argue that such activities were unprofessional, and called for error to be seen as anything that is a deviation from standard practice, thus protecting the health care system from infallibility. Mesman takes an interesting and novel approach to looking at patient safety, showing the work that goes into maintaining patient safety, as opposed to looking for and at error. Focusing on neo-natal care, she shows the intricate, almost orchestrated activities and efforts that go towards producing safe practice and care. Together these chapters look at the micro level of patient safety, albeit within a socio-cultural context, to better illustrate and explain how the day-to-day interactions that make up clinical practice produce a safe environment for patients and staff to accomplish their health care work.

In the theme of technology, Rowley shows how in the case of surgical instrumentation sometimes doing the 'wrong thing' can actually enhance patient safety under conditions of excessive risk or uncertainty. More broadly, it raises doubts over the commitment to guidelines and checklists as the panacea for unsafe clinical practice by showing how these can run counter to the realities of the clinical environment, expert judgement and notions of professionalism. Similarly, Pirnejad and Bal focus on the growth of information communication technologies, which are intended to lead to safer health care. Like Rowley however, they show

how technologies become shaped by or socialized into their particular practice and social environment, and can thus become unsafe or run counter the aspirations of patient safety. Together these chapters show how technologies become situated in practice, and as such, can be used in ways that are contrary to their intent and function, or in 'deviant' ways. Both chapters show how technologies aimed at enhancing patient safety can therefore create new risk and uncertainties in clinical practice that might not be anticipated by those who design and promote them.

In the theme of knowledge sharing, Waring and Currie lift the lid on adverse event incident reporting to surface the inherent politics that characterize attempts to foster learning and safety. Through exploring clinicians reactions and responses to reporting systems they question whether learning can truly be devoid of conflicting ideas, especially in relation to the enduring lines of power within health care organizations. Similarly, Bishop and Waring suggest that as an alternative to formal reporting systems lessons might be learnt from understanding how knowledge and experience are communicated within the informal communities and networks of health care. They show that in many instances problem-solving around patient safety events occurs rapidly and 'close to the action' through these organic communities and without recourse to formal reporting processes. Together these chapters suggest that the desire to improve communication in the wake of safety events and as a basis for learning might be more fruitful without the use of formal knowledge management systems, and instead service leaders should seek to harness those relationships and channels of communication that already exist.

Finally, in the theme of learning, Mengis and Nicolini's chapter extends these early discussions of knowledge sharing to consider what happens after incidents are reported, how they are investigated and how lessons are learnt. Focusing on the use of root cause analysis, they suggest learning remains an uneven and challenging task for health care organizations, despite the linear model of problem-solving advocated by its exponents. In particular, they show how such learning activities are undertaken in a complex social environment, characterized by recursive steps, negotiation and rapid change. Offering the possibility of additional models of learning and service improvement, Iedema's chapter highlights the role of action research and the way in which rapid service improvements can be made through embedding learning in practice. Together these chapters suggest the approach to learning typically portrayed within the patient safety literature fails to grasp the way social groups learn through 'doing' and that change might be better when learning is close to, or a part of, the action and not de-coupled from practice.

From the chapters offered in this collection we are able to identify a number of forgotten or marginal areas of theoretical and empirical inquiry that might provide a basis for future patient safety research. These are by no means exhaustive, nor do they necessarily reflect or represent the entire body of social sciences research that is currently being undertaken in the area of patient safety. However, they are areas of theory, research and practice that aim to move beyond the 'measure and manage' orthodoxy.

A Deeper Appreciation of Patient Safety

As pointed out above, a great deal of conceptual work has been made in rethinking the threats to patient safety, largely in terms of social psychology, ergonomics and human factors. This has been important for shifting attention away from individual errors to consider instead how these events are often conditioned or exacerbated by the wider system of work or latent factors (Reason 1997). Two interrelated questions are posed by this line of thinking. First, where should analysis stop, and second how can we understand the causal links between the system and the individual?

Although the human factors approach directs us to consider systemic factors, there is a tendency to focus on those factors located in the immediate work environment that influence cognitive performance and individual safety. It might be argued that this, in part, reflects the influence of social psychology in this 'systems' approach. It can also be seen, for example, in the application of root cause analysis where, as shown by Mengis and Nicolini, there is a tendency to focus on the local issues that can be 'fixed' rather than those wider system-level issues. Despite various elaborations and models that deconstruct 'the system' as a complex set of factors (for example Vincent 1997), there remains limited knowledge of how the wider organizational and institutional context influences safety. For example, major safety scandals consistently point to the role of regulatory systems in either encouraging or failing to protect against unsafe and dangerous practice, such as the Mid-Staffordshire Inquiry or the Shipman Inquiry (Smith 2004). In addition, research in other settings points to the way accidents can become an inevitable consequence of the way different organizational processes are 'coupled' (Perrow 1986) or how risks can become 'normalized' within prevailing cultures (Vaughan 1999). These ideas have only been applied at the margins of patient safety research to reveal, for example, how threats to safety in the operating department are brought about by the relationships between different hospital processes (Waring et al. 2006) and are often normalized by established professional cultures (Waring et al. 2007). A major under-researched issue, for instance, relates to the risks to safety found between care processes and organizations. This is an important area for research as the pathways and processes of patient care often cross community, primary and secondary care sectors, involving a variety of health and social care professionals, and might be better understood as a complex system. This is exemplified by the problems associated with hospital admission or discharge, or the long-term care of the elderly. So we might question therefore how 'deep' we want to take our analysis when thinking about the threats to patient safety, especially if we consider that some risks factors are indeed located deeper within the complex socio-cultural and political organization of health care systems.

If we take a deeper systems perspective, the question that follows is how best can we explain, even predict, the relationships between individual practice and the socio-cultural institutional environment? This is not simply about tracing error chains to find the links between causal factors: rather it relates to a long-standing problem for the social sciences encapsulated by the 'agency–structure' debate (for example Giddens 1984). Namely, do we seek to explain mistakes and risks in terms of wider social structures or rather as being located in the area of individual cognition and behaviour? Clearly, a systems approach moves beyond the individual towards some middle level, but how do we explain embedded patterns of action, cultures and ways of organizing? We might turn, for instance, to neo-institutional theory as found in organizational studies (Scott 1996). This provides a broad set of concepts and propositions to account for the patterns of organising social life, including regulatory, normative and cognitive-culture pillars. We might also consider a practice-based view of social action that focuses on the mediation of both agency and structure through routine social practice. The point is that we need to take a 'systems view' much more seriously, but when doing this we need find new or more appropriate theoretical and conceptual tools to help us explain the link between the unsafe system and unsafe practice.

The Positive, as well as the Negative, Dimensions of Patient Safety

Not only do we need a deeper understanding of the threats to patient safety, we might also benefit from a better appreciation of the positive, as well as negative factors that frame clinical practice and patient care. In line with the prevailing human factors approach, analytical attention has tended to centre on those latent factors that have a negative impact on service delivery and result in patient harm. Although statistics suggest that as many as one in ten patients experience some form of adverse event in their care (Department of Health 2000), and quite rightly we should seek to understand what brings about these events, we might also ask what makes for safe practice in the remaining 90 per cent of cases. Returning to the famous Swiss Cheese model, it might be argued that we have spent too much time looking for the holes and how to fill them, rather than looking for the cheese and how it can be replicated. We might advance patient safety through better recognizing and sharing the sources of safety in health care organizations. The work of Mesman is important in this regard because it highlights the resilience of health care professionals to maintain safety working conditions and tackle safety issues in their everyday practice. It highlights the often hidden or neglected work needed in maintaining patient safety that builds upon years of specialized training and clinical experience, as well as the informal routines and patterns that characterize local health care settings. As Palmer and Murcott suggest, however, attention to the positive aspects of patient safety, including safety innovations, is seemingly overshadowed by media and policy concern with what goes wrong!

This is not to suggest that the broad field of 'safety science' has neglected this issue: rather it appears that attention to the positive, as well as negative, might have been lost in the translation from industry to health care. Reason (1997), for instance, describes organizations as existing within and moving through safety 'space'. This space is portrayed as something like a spectrum of safety characteristics and latent factors, some of which are inherently positive and others negative.

From this perspective, organizations are challenged with navigating the safety space through utilizing available risk management and learning systems, such as incident reporting. However, it might be argued that too often these navigational tools focus on learning from failure rather than success. Future research is needed therefore to understand, not only the sources of safety and resilience in clinical practice, but also how more systematic means of identifying and sharing these lessons might be developed. This might include, for instance, harnessing those professional networks and communities of practice that characterize day-to-day clinical services. As shown by Bishop and Waring, these provide a powerful basis for sharing information, enabling problem-solving and ultimately producing safety close to the action. Although these might not engender the type of system-wide or organizational learning envisaged by policies, they do make an important contribution to patient safety and should not be ignored in the pursuit to establish more formal navigational tools, such as incident reporting.

Moreover, we need to be cautious about thinking that what might look like unsafe or deviant practice is always a threat to patient safety. Rowley shows, for example, that breaking the rules can be an important act in maintaining or assuring safety in the context of wider perceived risks. More broadly, there is a tendency to associate safety with rule-following and a belief that checklists and protocols are the answers to correcting, limiting or inhibiting deviant or unsafe practice (Gawande 2010). Here much attention is given to the contribution of checklists in the aviation industry, in the use of heavy machinery and, increasingly, in the operating theatre. However, this again tends to focus on the micro or local level of patient safety, especially the immediate environmental or team conditions that lead to cognitive disruptions and behaviour errors. These are clearly essential issues to be considered and addressed, but by focusing on these, we run the risk of downplaying or ignoring that the deeper 'latent' sources of risk might be institutional or organizational in origin. Moreover, the use of rules and checklists can be too prescriptive. It often neglects that health care is a highly complex, non-linear system and that assuring safe working in one particular environment or silo still relies upon assuring the safety in other connected processes. It also downplays the fact that professional practice needs to be able to recognize and cope with uncertainty and complexity. Conformity to rules or checklists can foster learned helplessness or undermine the capacity of professionals to identify and tackle uncertain working conditions that are not prescribed by the rules (McDonald et al. 2006). It might be suggested therefore that patient safety research look beyond the obvious sources of safety as found in other sectors, and spend more time understanding the sources of resilience and safety that already exist in day-to-day clinical practice.

Emotion and Patient Safety

Although patient safety events have significant, even fatal consequences for patients, they also have profound implications for clinicians. Mistakes, mishaps and adverse incidents represent major psychological and emotional events for those involved. Clinicians may feel, for instance, not only sadness or guilt for harm caused, but also self-doubt and a loss of confidence. Although systems of professional education have long been recognized as providing both informal and formal mechanisms for acknowledging and managing the psychosocial aspects of clinical practice (Bosk 1979, Stephenson et al. 2001), there remains little contemporary research exploring the links between patient safety and emotion; either how safety events impact upon the emotions of clinicians, or how emotions affect how clinicians engage in safety practices.

By far the most prominent emotional consideration within the current body of safety research relates to the issue of 'blame' (Department of Health 2000). As described elsewhere in this collection, this blame culture is seen as stemming from a lack of attention to the latent factors that bring about clinical risk and a continued focus on individual behaviour and conduct (Reason 2000). Over the last decade strenuous efforts have been made to foster 'systems thinking' and cultural change, often making reference to the importance of 'psychological safety' in improving communication and learning (Edmondson 1999). However, blame remains only one emotional response to patient safety events. It can be anticipated that clinicians might also feel sadness, regret and surprise when safety events occur. Paget (1988), for example, described medical culture as being characterized by a 'complex sorry' whereby clinicians' retrospective assessment of their performance reflects a desire that events may have turned out differently. Research also shows that emotions related to patient safety in terms of decision making (Croskerry et al. 2010), teamwork (Nurkok et al. 2011) and participation in reporting systems (Waring et al. 2010). Moreover, Mengis and Nicolini's chapter shows the emotional work involved in investigating incidents.

In terms of developing research in this area a number of possible lines of enquiry can be suggested. First, efforts should be made, not only to tackle the problem of blame, but also to recognize and understand the complex emotional responses to patient safety events. These might have wide-ranging, often unanticipated effects for clinicians that extend beyond the workplace and include prolonged periods of staff sickness and absence. Second, we need to understand more about how service leaders can develop emotional intelligence (Mayer et al. 2008) or their ability to recognize and manage the emotions of their staff. Too often this is an assumed skill, but more attention should be given to developing this amongst service leaders.

Safety and Productivity

A final observation relates to potential tensions and difficulties of balancing productivity and safety. Although safety has been a major policy priority for at least ten years, during much of this time we have seen record levels of investment in health care services. In the wake of the global financial crisis in 2008 and in context of reduced public spending, health care services around the world need to make efficiency savings, especially in largely publicly financed and provided systems such as the UK NHS. As such we are seeing increased attention to approaches and methodologies, such as lean thinking, that promise to delivery efficiency saving and enhance productivity, whilst at the same time delivering quality and safety (Womack and Jones 2003).

With its origins in the Toyota Production Systems (TPS), 'lean thinking' has become particularly popular (Womack and Jones 2003, Liker 2004). Central to its philosophy is a concern with waste – *muda* – or processes that add no value to the product or customer. This waste is elaborated in seven areas, including transportation, inventory, motion, waiting, overproduction, over processing and defects. To reduce this waste, five principles of 'lean thinking' are proposed. The first is to specify the 'value' created by the operational process. This should not be dominated by provider interests, but instead should reflect what the customer will value. The second involves identifying 'value streams' or those processes that will ultimately add value to the product. This can be achieved through forms of problem-solving and change management, often through re-drawing activities that add value, whilst eliminating those that do not. The third involves creating 'flow' throughout these processes. This means breaking down the boundaries and divisions between organizational and occupational groups to ensure work streams are continually attuned to the creation of value. The fourth highlights the importance of demand or 'pull' through responding to the needs of customers, rather than suppliers. And finally, it strives for 'perfection' or the idea that 'lean thinking' should be a continuous activity embedded within the culture of the organisation.

Over the last decade process re-engineering methodologies have been applied widely across the public and health care service (Institute for Health Improvement 2005, Zidel 2006, NHS Confederation 2006, Proudlove et al. 2008, Radnor and Boaden 2008, Young and McClean 2008). Research also shows the potential benefits of service reconfiguration to patient care and resource utilization (Kim et al. 2005, Jones and Filochowski 2006, Joosten et al. 2009). At a philosophical and methodological level, approaches such as lean thinking actually reflect and align with those of the patient safety agenda. They both aim to identify system-level factors that result in error or remedial steps, which in turn produce both waste and patient harm. However, research also shows that the implementation of lean thinking is not without its problems, with the process depending on factors such as organizational readiness, a culture of continuous improvement, effective leadership, the availability of resources and communication strategy (Radnor and Boaden 2008). Moreover, in practice lean thinking involves considerable variability, with some services adopting a system-wide approach, whilst others tentatively adopt specific techniques from the lean thinking toolbox (Burgess et al. 2009).

It is also worth reflecting that the balance between productivity and safety is not always easy to achieve. Even Toyota has struggled to simultaneously maintain both demands, as exemplified by the safety problems and major recalls between

2009 and 2011 (National Highway Traffic Safety Administration 2010). Health care providers who embark on implementing lean thinking or other such process re-engineering activities, need to continually ensure that they are delivering quality and safety as well as enhancing productivity. One line of research might be to explore the synergies between these agendas and integrate the different models for delivery safety and productivity – after all, they are not mutually exclusive. One issue for example, might relate to the tendency of health services to apply lean thinking at the local or micro level through a series of quick-fixes or 'low-hanging fruit' (Radnor and Boaden 2008, Burgess et al. 2009, Radnor et al. in press). This means that many of the wider system-level issues that affect productivity might be overlooked. This clearly has strong parallels with the theory of 'systems thinking' as found in the patient safety literature, even if research and practice sometime neglect this wider system component. As such, there is a clear case for integrating systems thinking with lean thinking to ensure that productivity improvements are widespread and substantial, but also directed at improving operational safety.

The Future?

Our collection aims to advance, not detract from, the enormously important advances made in the area of patient safety research and practice. Although it might appear, at time, critical of the efforts and advance in scholarship made by the world's leading patient safety researchers and exponents, its ultimate intent is to suggest that the promotion of patient safety might benefit from additional, and not always complementary, ways of thinking. Just like those early researchers who worked to highlight the mistakes and errors of health care delivery and to promote the importance of a new, 'systems' approach to patient safety, the chapters in this collection argue that we might also need to go further and take a more full account of the complex socio-cultural context that frames health care work and organization. The future requires more connections and collaborations between ideas and more interdisciplinary research. In conclusion, we hope this collection stimulates critical thinking: critical in the sense that is offers a counterpoint or alternative to approaches and methodologies that have themselves become an orthodoxy, and also in the belief that these socio-cultural perspective are of critical importance if we are serious about improving patient safety.

References

Bosk, C. 1979. *Forgive and Remember: Managing Medical Mistakes*, Chicago: Chicago University Press.
Brennan, T.A., Leape, L.L., Laird, N.M., Hebert, L., Localio, A.R., Lawthers, A.G., Newhouse, J.P., Weiler, P.C. and Hiatt, H.H. 1991. Incidence of adverse events and negligence in hospitalized patients. Results of the Harvard Medical Practice Study I, *New England Journal of Medicine*, 324(6), 370–6.

Burgess, N., Radnor, Z. and Davies, R. 2009. Taxonomy of lean in health care: a framework for evaluating activity and impact. Paper presented at the EUROMA Conference, Sweden.

Croskerry, P., Abbass, A. and Wu, A. 2010. Emotional influences in patient safety, *Journal of Patient Safety*, 6(4), 199–205.

Department of Health. 2000. *An Organisation with a Memory*, London: TSO.

Edmonson, A. 1999. Psychological safety and learning behaviours in work teams, *Administrative Science Quarterly*, 44(2), 350–83.

Gawande, A. 2010. *The Checklist Manifesto*, New York: Henry Holt and Co.

Giddens, A. 1984. *The Constitution of Society*, Cambridge: Polity Press.

Institute for Health Improvement. 2005. *Going Lean in Healthcare*, Cambridge, Institute for Health Improvement.

Institute of Medicine. 1999. *To Err is Human: Building A Safer Health System*, Washington: National Academy Press.

Jones, D. and Filochowski, J. 2006. Lean health care. Think yourself thin, *Health Services Journal*, 1116(Apr), s6–7.

Joosten, T., Bongers, I. and Janssen, R. 2009. The application of lean to health care: issues and observations, *Quality and Safety in Healthcare*, 21(5), 341–7.

Kim, C., Spahlinger, D., Kin, J. and Billi, J. 2005. Lean health care: what hospitals can learn from a world class auto-maker, *Journal of Hospital Medicine*, 1(3), 191–9.

Leape, L.L. 1997. A systems analysis to medical error, *Journal of Evaluation in Clinical Practice*, 3(3), 213–22.

Liker, J. 2004. *The Toyota Way*, Madison: McGraw-Hill.

Lilford, R. 2010. The English Patient Safety Research Programme: a commissioner's tale, *Journal of Health Services Research and Policy*, 15(supp.1), 1–3.

Mayer, J.D., Salovey, P. and Caruso, D.R. 2008. Emotional intelligence: new ability or eclectic traits, *American Psychologist*, 63(6), 503–17.

McDonald, R., Waring, J. and Harrison, S. 2006. Clinical guidelines, patient safety and the narrativisation of identity: an operating department case study, *Sociology of Health and Illness*, 28(2), 178–202.

NHS Confederation. 2006. *Lean Thinking for the NHS*, London: NHS Confederation.

National Highway Traffic Safety Administration. 2010. *U.S. Department of Transportation Responds to Third Toyota Recall*. Online source: http://www.nhtsa.gov/PR/DOT-25-10 (accessed 3rd May 2011).

Nurkok, M., Lipsitz, S. Satwicz, P., Kelly, A. and Frankel, A. 2011. A novel method for reproducibly measuring the effects of interventions to improve emotional climate, indices of team skills and communication, and the threat to patient outcome in high-volume thoracic surgery center, *Archive of Surgery*, 145(5), 489–97.

Paget, M.A. 1988. *The Unity of Mistakes: A Phenomenological Interpretation of Medical Work*, Philadelphia: Temple University Press.

Perrow, C. 1986. *Normal Accidents: Living with High Risk Technologies*, New York: Princeton University Press.

Proudlove, N., Moxham, C. and Boaden, R. 2008. Lessons for lean in health care from using six sigma in the NHS, *Public Money and Management*, February, 27–34.

Radnor, Z. and Boaden, R. 2008. Lean in the public services: panacea or paradox? *Public Money and Management*, 28(1), 3–6.

Radnor, Z., Holweg, M. and Waring, J. (in press) Lean health care: an unfulfilled promise? *Social Science and Medicine*, http://www.sciencedirect.com/science/article/pii/S0277953611000979.

Reason, J. 1997. *Managing the Risks of Organizational Accidents*, Aldershot: Ashgate.

Reason, J. 2000. Human error: models and management, *British Medical Journal*, 320(7237), 768–70.

Scott, R. 1996. *Institutions and Organizations*, London: Sage.

Smith, J. (Chair). 2004. *The Shipman Inquiry Fifth Report – Safeguarding Patients: Lessons from the Past, Proposals for the Future*, London: TSO.

Stephenson, A., Higgs, R. and Sugarman, J. 2001. Teaching professional development in medical schools, *The Lancet*, 375(9259), 876–70.

Vaughan, D. 1999. The dark side of organizations: mistakes, misconduct, disaster, *Annual Review of Sociology*, 25, 271–305.

Vincent, C. and Reason, J. 1999. Human factors approaches in medicine. In: *Medical Mishaps*, edited by M. Rosenthal, L. Mulcahy and S. Lloyd-Bostock, Buckingham: Open University Press, pp. 39–56.

Vincent, C. 1997. Risk, safety and the dark side of quality, *British Medical Journal*, 314, 175.

Waring, J., McDonald, R. and Harrison, S. 2006. Safety and complexity: the inter-departmental threats to patient safety in the operating department, *Journal of Health, Organisation and Management*, 20(3), 227–42.

Waring, J., Harrison, S. and McDonald, R. 2007. A culture of safety or coping: ritualistic behaviours in the operating department, *Journal of Health Services Research and Policy*, 12(1), supp. 1, 3.

Waring, J., Rowley, E., Dingwall, R., Palmer, C. and Murcott, T. 2010. A narrative review of the UK Patient Safety Research Portfolio, *Journal of Health Services Research and Policy*, 15(1), supp. 2, 26–32.

Womack, J. and Jones, D. 2003. *Lean Thinking*, London: Simon & Schuster.

Young, T. and McClean, S. 2008. A critical look at lean thinking in health care, *Quality and Safety in Health Care*, 17, 382–6.

Zidel, T. 2006. *A Lean Guide To Transforming Healthcare*, Milwaukee: ASQ.

... ...

Index